The Finger

WITHDRAWN

ALSO BY ANGUS TRUMBLE

A Brief History of the Smile

The Finger

A HANDBOOK

Angus Trumble

YALE UNIVERSITY PRESS

LONDON

This edition published in the United Kingdom by Yale University Press
Printed in the United Kingdom by TJ International Ltd, Padstow, Cornwall

Illustration credits appear on pages xi–xvi.

A catalogue record for this book is available from the British Library

ISBN 978-0-300-16666-8 (hardcover : alk. paper)

Designed by Jonathan D. Lippincott

www.yalebooks.co.uk

1   3   5   7   9   10   8   6   4   2

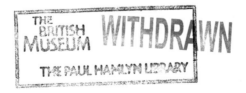

In memory of my mother,

Helen Trumble

ESSE QUAM VIDERI

Turner's palm is as itchy as his fingers are ingenious.
—Sir Walter Scott to his friend
the artist James Skene, April 30, 1823

The white hand like a lady's, with taper fingers and filbert nails, delicately tinged with rose-color, that guided the inspired pen from midnight until midday, was never aching and cramped.
—"Temple Bar" on Honoré de Balzac,
The New York Times, January 5, 1879

The artist, like the God of creation, remains within or behind or beyond or above his handiwork, invisible, refined out of existence, indifferent, paring his fingernails.
—James Joyce, *A Portrait of the Artist as a Young Man*, 1916

Contents

List of Illustrations

A Note on Finger Numbering and Terminology

Most writers and cultures agreed that the five fingers could be counted in one of two ways: (a) beginning with the thumb and proceeding to the little finger, or (b) beginning with the index finger, proceeding in the same direction as before, and ending with the thumb. The problem is brought out at the beginning of the long and fascinating article in the *Oxford English Dictionary* where *finger* is defined as "one of the five terminal members of the hand; in a restricted sense, one of the four excluding the thumb. In this latter sense, the fingers are commonly numbered first to fourth, starting from that next the thumb [the index finger]."

Among the numerous authorities that immediately follow, the frequently cited *South English Legendary* (c. 1280–90) mentions that the devil has "fif [five] fyngres"; in other words: Beware, he might easily look like you or me. Meanwhile, a fifteenth-century source refers to the "thowmbe" as the "fyfte fynger." However, the matrimonial rubric of Archbishop Thomas Cranmer's *Book of Common Prayer* (1549) explicitly states that the ring will be placed on the "fowerth finger of the womans left hand," which implies numbering from the thumb onward.

This matter vexed the otherwise unflappable New Zealander R. W. Burchfield in "finger," his brief article in the revised third edition of *Fowler's Modern English Usage* (1998). He follows the *OED*: "The fingers are now usually numbered exclusively of the thumb—*first* (or *fore* or *index*), *second* (or *middle*), *third* (or *ring*), and *fourth* (or *little*); but in the marriage service the third is called the fourth. It is also the fourth in the modern method of indicating the fingering of keyboard music, in which the thumb, formerly marked *x*, is now 1, and the fingers are numbered correspondingly."

Fortunately, as far as I can see, these are the only two numbering systems that have ever existed, and while it is often unclear, especially in the rich eighteenth- and nineteenth-century antiquarian literature on finger rings, for example, which of them applies, almost always the ring finger (next to the little finger) provides a reliable key to identifying the rest because the ancient custom of wearing the wedding ring on that one either antedates or at least overrides them both. As Dean Comber correctly explained, in that finger "the ancients thought there was a vein that came directly from the heart."

At any rate, choosing between these two methods of numbering the fingers generally reflects a vague assumption about whether or not the thumb may be defined as a bona fide finger. Certainly few have ever proposed counting in the opposite direction, starting with the little finger, and one wonders why such a strategy should now strike us as perverse. A noteworthy exception to this rule is Plato, who, in *The Republic*, has Socrates showing three of his fingers to the hapless Glaucon in an effort to develop his important (and happy) distinction between the visible and the intelligible—not always fully grasped these days by art historians, curators, critics, and museum professionals. "Here, we say," says Socrates, "are three fingers, the little finger, the second, and the middle." The order is not explicitly stated, but since the little and middle fingers are clearly identified, it follows that Socrates' "second" finger is the ring, not the index.

The only other example I have found of counting the fingers in this manner, beginning with the little finger, occurs obliquely in a discussion of the natural path of human life by Christopher Ness in his *Compleat History and Mystery of the Old*

and New Testament. This, he says, "we may learn from our fingers' ends, the dimensions [i.e., lengths] whereof demonstrate
this to us, beginning with the end of the little finger, representing our childhood, rising up to a little higher at the end of the
ring-finger, which betokens our youth; from it to the top of the
middle finger, which is the highest point of our elevated hand,
and so most aptly represents our middle age, when we come
to our acme, or height of stature and strength; then begins our
declining age, from thence to the end of our forefinger, which
amounts to a little fall, but from thence to the end of the thumb
there is a great fall, to shew, when man goes down in his old age,
he falls fast and far ..."

On the whole, however, when they are deployed for allegor-
ical or mnemonic purposes, finger sequences run in the opposite
direction, as in Ben Jonson's *The Alchemist*, where "The thumb,
in chiromancy, we give to Venus, / The fore-finger to Jove; the
midst to Saturn; / The ring to Sol; the least to Mercury," and
likewise most European languages continue to take their cue
from the Latin *digitus primus* ("first finger," i.e., thumb), modern conventions of musical keyboard notation, and the scientific
community, for whom the thumb is D[igit]1 or I, the index finger D2 or II, and so on down to D5/DV, the little finger.

Throughout this book I have numbered the fingers accord-
ingly and, except where the specific terms and their variants are
under review, including

pollex	*demonstratorius*	*impudicus*	*annularis*	*auricularis*
	scite-finger	*medius*	annular finger	ear-finger
	fore-finger	*famosus*	gold-finger	pink, or pinky
	trigger finger	*obscenus*	medical finger	little man
	foreman	longman	physic finger	
	toucher	middle-man	leche-man	
		long finger	leech-finger	
		fool's finger		

of which a few are still in common use, especially *fore-finger*, I have named each consistently as follows:

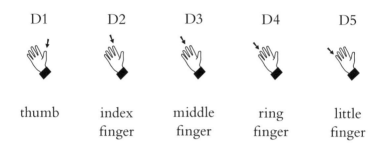

D1	D2	D3	D4	D5
thumb	index finger	middle finger	ring finger	little finger

The Finger

ONE

The Finger: A Few Pointers

He has ears, and two eyes, and ten fingers,
Leastways if you reckon two thumbs;
Long ago he was one of the singers,
But now he is one of the dumbs.

—from Edward Lear, "How Pleasant
to Know Mr. Lear!" 1879

In *Middlemarch*, George Eliot bequeathed to future generations the sobering example of the Reverend Mr. Casaubon, that "great bladder for dried peas to rattle in!" as Mrs. Cadwallader so memorably described him—a warning, in other words, against too ambitious or arid a scholarly enterprise, and too hopeless a quest for comprehensiveness. So while using my own fingers to write this book, I have from time to time experienced a sinking feeling that it might too closely resemble an absurd *Key to All Mythologies*. In those gloomy moments, I have paused for a cup of tea and tried to focus instead on the beautiful, and in our culture fortunately still flourishing, seventeenth- and eighteenth-century ideal of the essay, which, at least in its French derivation, means nothing more than "a try," a stab at it, a particular view at a given moment, a series of reflections that, by cutting deeply enough into (in this case) one narrow seam of human anatomy and experience, may with luck provide access to rather more.

So while this book contains a lot of information that may be useful for future inquirers about fingers and finger lore, I hope that it will give at least some pleasure and food for thought to nonspecialist readers in what we have conveniently come to know as the digital age. Nevertheless, the *handbook* portion of my title is a genuine aspiration, and it may be of some comfort to the reader in search of specific technical, historical, cultural, or other folkloric references that while, for obvious reasons, *The Finger: A Handbook* shuns footnotes, I have instead attempted to provide as much documentation as possible in the endnotes.

My last book, *A Brief History of the Smile*, began its life as a lecture at a conference of dentists. *The Finger: A Handbook* owes its existence to a similar collision between the world of art museums (in which I have made my career) and the medical profession. In 1998, a group of orthopedic surgeons in Adelaide, South Australia, led by Dr. Michael Hayes, invited me to give a talk at a conference about hand injuries. For this group, whose interests and activities were far more varied than those of the dentists, I proposed a talk about a particular gesture of the right hand, a pointing gesture. It is common enough, the index finger extended; the middle, ring, and little fingers folded onto the palm; and while the thumb is not necessarily held in along the side of the folded middle finger, or against the outer edge of the index finger, nor is it generally extended as far as possible, as in a child's worrying approximation of a loaded pistol. The specific, ancient Roman meaning of this more disciplined pointing gesture has today been largely forgotten, yet it crops up in many places.

In the courtyard of the Palazzo dei Conservatori in Rome, one may still see a disembodied right hand of this type, one of a number of fragments of a colossal marble statue of Emperor Constantine the Great (324–37 C.E.). In its present position, the enormous index finger points straight up. The expatriate Swiss artist Henry Fuseli was so moved by the scale of these pieces of

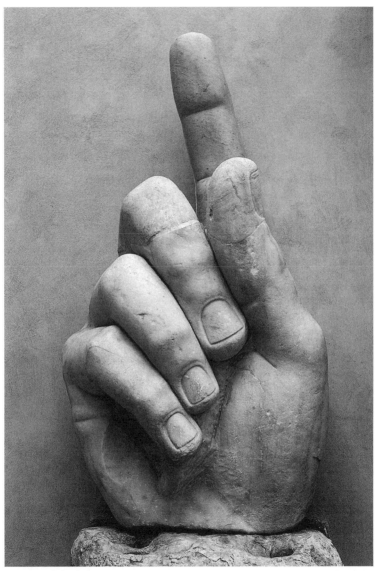

Much fortified by its usefulness in Roman rhetoric and "oratorical delivery," the index finger, in this case that of Constantine the Great, was also a potent emblem of military command.

marble—and the imagined magnificence of the vanished statue to which they once belonged—that he drew himself dwarfed by the stone hand, cradling his head in his own, the left. He called the drawing *The Artist Moved to Despair by the Grandeur of Antique Fragments*. This was in the years 1778–80, and Fuseli's fantasy self-portrait drawing has since become a popular and enduring symbol of European Romanticism. The most famous intact example of this ancient Roman gesture is that of the emperor Augustus, whose Prima Porta statue was one of the greatest archaeological discoveries of the nineteenth century (1863) and is now in the Braccio Nuovo of the Vatican Museums. His arm raised, Augustus makes the very same pointing gesture with his right hand.

Close by, on the ceiling of the Sistine Chapel (1508–12), Michelangelo Buonarroti brilliantly represented the account in Genesis of the creation of man by means of two proximate gestures of the hand. The ingenious sense of drama with which the artist prevented the fingers of those two powerful hands from touching—the hand of God the Father with the pointing index finger, and the awakening hand of Adam, his left—gives the image its emotional charge. No wonder many people read the tiny intervening space as filled with energy, traversed by a powerful aesthetic "zap." The junction of these two magnificent hands, the one brimming with energy, the other with incipient life, is endlessly reproduced as a detail—these days in advertisements for electrical goods or financial services. We tend to see it as magical, animating, supremely eloquent. But there is good evidence to suggest that the gesture with which God the Father summons Adam into being is not magical so much as military, at the very least commanding in flavor, specifically a gesture of command generally associated with Roman emperors such as Augustus and Constantine, and generals upon whom imperial authority devolved in the field. Its meaning was well understood. Supported by angels, God commands man into corporeal existence: "Be!"

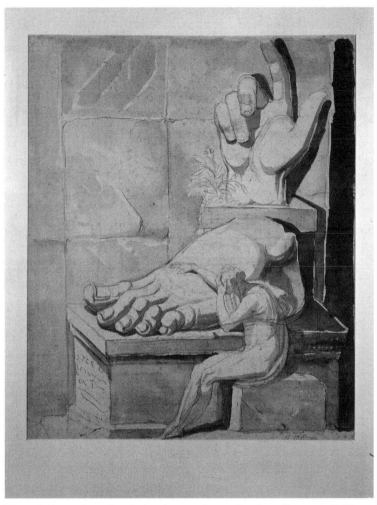

Though "moved to despair by the grandeur of antique fragments," Henry Fuseli evidently felt free to modify the disposition of the colossal digits, and relax them.

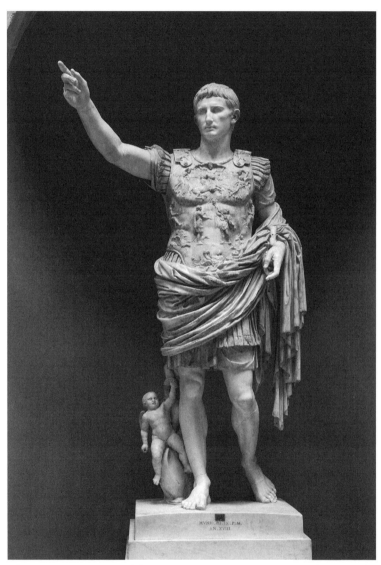

The Prima Porta statue of the emperor Augustus provides a useful model for how the fragmentary hand of Constantine may have been joined to the original statue. The gesture is, of course, the same.

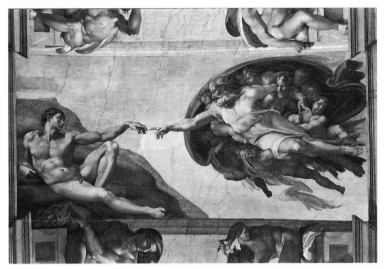

As a set piece of pictorial drama, Michelangelo's depiction of the creation of man on the ceiling of the Sistine Chapel turns upon the fulcrum of the converging index fingers of Adam and God.

Comparatively few of us employ our fingers as instruments of command, but everyone uses them to indicate. Indeed, for the infant pointing is an indispensable tool for the miraculous acquisition of language itself. But the fundamental act of pointing at people and things is only the beginning. Our fingers ultimately follow in gesture many syntactical trajectories. In his great 1632 group portrait of doctors observing an anatomical dissection, *The Anatomy of Dr. Nicolaes Tulp* (1632), Rembrandt chose as the focus of the composition the moment when Dr. Tulp takes up with his forceps certain tendons of the cadaver's forearm. Those tendons were (correctly) thought to help produce the opposition of the thumb and index finger—that single most important physical asset that has made it possible for us to ascend to our present position at the top of the evolutionary tree. It is rare to find a work of art that pays such tribute to the exact motor functions of the index finger and thumb, though, of course, it is precisely those that painters rely on, and rely on completely, when they tackle the complicated task of picture making. Rembrandt further emphasized the specific meaning of the subject, because with his own free left hand Dr. Tulp offers a vivid demonstration of the physical mechanism of the same tendons he holds with the forceps in his right.

Unlike Rembrandt, most artists have been content to exploit the full range of gestures of which our hands and fingers are capable, to which generations of observers have willingly attached an enormous range of meanings over the centuries. One thinks of the German Renaissance *Isenheim Altarpiece* by Matthias Grünewald, that terrifying portrayal of the crucifixion of Jesus Christ in which an out-of-time St. John the Baptist, that powerful presence in the opening verses of the Gospel of John, "bears witness" to the light by pointing at Jesus' dying body with the elongated, outstretched, tautly upward-sloping, tapering index finger of his right hand.

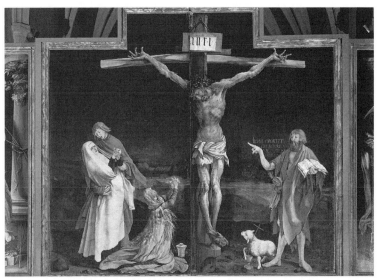

Indication, suffering, supplication, and despair: in his *Isenheim Altarpiece*, Matthias Grünewald exploited to the fullest extent the expressive and narrative potential of the fingers.

John's gesture is as controlled as the carefully articulated fingers of the expiring Christ, extending from mutilated palms at the summit of the altarpiece, writhe and curl and twitch in agony. In doing so, they carry for Grünewald a considerable part of the heavy burden of the baffling, mystical narrative of the cross: the instrument of torture, the tree of life. To the left, John, the beloved disciple, supports the Virgin Mary, his slender fingers trained gingerly around her waist, while St. Mary Magdalene, kneeling at the foot of the cross, raises her clasped hands, the fingers tightly intertwined but straight, stiffened by hot grief and dismay, a fervent gesture that contrasts sharply with the folded hands of Jesus' fainting mother.

Some of the earliest of all surviving man-made images are of fingers—the silhouettes of disembodied hands with spreading fingers that adorn the walls of caves and other rock shelters in Spain and France and China and Australia. The artist simply placed his hand against the rock, fingers splayed, then took a mouthful of paint, and blew a fine spray over the back of the hand and the immediately surrounding rock surface. When the hand was lifted off, a ghostly "negative" image remained—the earliest form of printing. Primitive man knew perfectly well that the image he produced by this method was far more durable and accurate than the poorer substitute produced by dipping the hand in paint and applying a handprint. Thin coatings of paint, sprayed from the mouth, adhere better and last longer than thicker ones applied under pressure, which tend to crack and peel off.

In a surprisingly large number of examples there are parts of fingers missing or distinctly shortened, possibly the grisly evidence of Ice Age frostbite, or else some form of prehistoric ritual mutilation, scarification, or punishment. In some places there are dozens of these spectral hands and fingers; elsewhere only one has survived. It has occasionally been suggested that prehistoric hand images in caves and rock shelters that apparently lack one

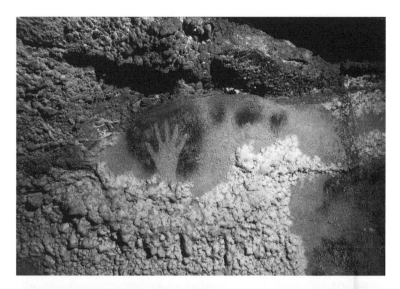

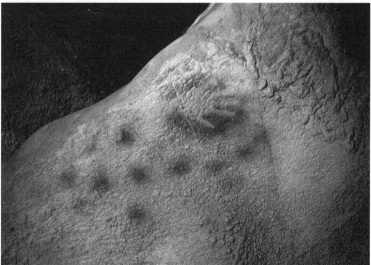

These hand silhouettes in the Grotte de Pech Merle at Cabrerets (Lot) in France were made between 15,000 and 14,000 years before the Common Era; similar images survive in caves and rock shelters elsewhere in France, as well as in Spain, China, and Australia.

or two of the outermost finger joints or, at times, whole fingers, are in fact the result of folding under the relevant digit and
spraying over the hand configured so as to deploy one of a range
of carefully differentiated signs with particular meaning. While
it may never be possible to rule out this possibility, the available
photographic evidence suggests that this is unlikely to be true.
      It is not physically possible to fold double only the terminal
bone or "phalanx" of any finger. This would be necessary to produce those images in which only that phalanx is missing. When
a film of paint is sprayed over an object of relatively consistent
depth that is placed flat against a supporting surface, any variation in depth such as one might expect to observe in a hand
placed flat against a stone but with one finger (or more) folded
under will tend to produce in the resulting silhouette a corresponding variation in the consistency of line. By the technique
of spraying paint from the mouth, the outline of a folded finger
ought to be fuzzier and less distinct than the crisper outline of
its outstretched neighbors. As far as I can tell, this is not generally
the case. Prehistoric hand and finger silhouettes are remarkably
even in outline. Either they genuinely preserve the profile of a
hand with partly missing digits, or the image was tampered with
or "corrected" after the initial spraying so as to adjust the outline
for clarity.
      Why are these mysterious prehistoric relics so moving? It
is not merely their extreme antiquity. It is also, I think, the fact
that they correspond so exactly with what most of us now observe projecting fussily from the end of each arm—every day,
all day long, the only parts of our bodies, moreover, that we
see (without the aid of mirrors) routinely uncovered, acceptably
naked. Today we might expect to create an almost identical imprint with our own hands were we to follow those simple steps,
and indeed, until recently some Australian Aborigines still added
their handprint to that chorus of ancestors with whom they
cherish an unbroken connection. This is humbling.

That constant visual engagement with our own hands and fingers, often at extremely close range, can have unexpected consequences. Beginning in 1958, the British Broadcasting Corporation aired a series of television programs entitled *Your Life in Their Hands*, which was all about surgery. This was not for the fainthearted, because a number of these presented whole operations, benefiting from what was still in Australia the relatively recent introduction of color television, in graphic close-up. As a schoolboy, I remember being fascinated and far from repelled by most episodes. There was mostly an abstract quality to that tightly circumscribed rectangle of sanitized operating-theater green cotton which placed at one remove the untidy jumble of shiny pink organs wobbling inside the tummy or chest cavity. One saw the surgeon forthrightly thrusting his gloved hands inside, rummaging for arteries, extracting tumors, then sewing the whole thing up with a needle and thread. There was in this spectacle a detached quality that for the layman made it not merely tolerable, but at times engrossing too.

Only one of these programs, I recall, induced a certain clamminess in the palms of the hands and sharp intakes of breath, and eventually caused me to change channels. This dealt with an operation on the tendons of somebody's hand. There is something particularly desperate about seeing the surgeon's scalpel gain entry to a part of the body that is as constantly before one's eyes as a thumb or finger. In that sense only, it is impossible to place at arm's length. Which makes you wince more readily, the thought of hitting the top of your head on a low beam, developing acute appendicitis, or by accident getting your finger jammed in a door? "Men's natures wrangle with inferior things, / Though great ones are their object . . ." says Desdemona. "For let our finger ache, and it indues / Our other healthful members even to that sense / Of pain."

From the earliest days of our infancy we rely upon our fingers to explore, then navigate through, a gradually loosening confinement in space, and to reach vital conclusions about temperature, motion, texture, weight, sharpness, hardness—in other words, about practically everything our eyes and ears cannot yet comprehend. In the evolution of language, it comes as no surprise therefore to find that finger words, expressions, and sayings are extremely ancient.

The long migration of the English words *finger* and *thumb* commences even before the advent of Old English (where they had already assumed the familiar forms of *fynger* and *thuma*). They had solidified already in the Gothic, Old Teutonic, even apparently pre-Teutonic languages (extending far back into antiquity, as far as we can tell from those few texts that have insured their survival in one form or another). Thenceforth, both words found their way into Old Frisian, Old Swedish, Old High German, Old Norse, and other archaic languages. Thence they descended to our northern European cousin languages, which still retain essentially the same word: *Finger* and *Daumen* (in German); *vinger* and *duim* (Dutch); *finger* but interestingly *tommelfinger* (Danish); *finger* and *tumme* (Swedish); and so on. It seems likely that the pre-Teutonic origin of *finger* is somehow bound to the simple concept of five, while I suppose for obvious, if somewhat gloomy reasons the word *thumb* owes its existence to the idea of shortness, stoutness, or "wanting."

In fact, the gradual accretion of finger words, expressions, and sayings in English seems to have occurred in connection with a few highly specific concepts, including measurement (a finger's breadth), resemblance (dead men's fingers, fish fingers), skill (having a green thumb, or nimble fingers), precision (snapping the fingers), desire (itchy fingers), concision (thumbnail sketch), clumsiness (all thumbs), slightness of motion (to stir or lift a finger), manipulation in its sinister sense, and theft. And it is surprising to find just how many of these are apparently distasteful. True, we keep our fingers crossed for luck, and when at times we succeed in grasping an idea we may say we *put our finger on it*.

If, with luck, that idea stayed with us, we may once have boasted that we had it *at our fingers' ends*, or nowadays *at our fingertips*. In *Pamela* (1740), Samuel Richardson mentioned that Miss L——— has "an admirable finger upon the harpsichord." In other words, she played well. It was said of the English actor George Arliss (1868–1946) that he could "express more with one finger than most actors can express with their entire bodies."

The fingers certainly offer convenient opportunities for nicely crafted superlatives, which even crop up in the Hebrew Bible, where "my little finger shall be thicker than my father's loins," and often in Shakespeare ("Thy hand is but a finger to my fist"). But for each of these, there is a host of less attractive concepts for which the fingers have clearly provided a suitable metaphor. In *Troilus and Cressida*, mention is made of "the devil Luxury, with his fat rump and potato-finger." And among the ingredients of the witches' cauldron in *Macbeth*, perhaps the most revolting is "Finger of birth-strangled babe, ditch-deliver'd by a drab."

No doubt this vulnerability to pejorative usage is at least partly due to the persistent idea, originating with Aristotle, that the sense of touch is comparatively "dark," or at least lower in rank than sight, hearing, smell, and taste—in that order. To Aristotle the sense of touch was the most basic of all the senses, indeed the only one common to all animals. As Cynthia Freeland has observed, the fact that certain creatures such as barely animate sponges seemed to possess the sense of touch alone, and none of the others, was sufficient to distinguish them from the apparently senseless plants that they so closely resemble. Perhaps because of its innateness, indeed complexity, Aristotle saw touch as far more fundamentally linked to certain biological and bodily processes, such as eating, drinking, having sex, going to sleep, growing old, getting sick, and dying than the other, "higher" senses, even though vision and hearing demonstrably wobble and diminish as a more or less direct result of any one of these phenomena.

In his *De anima*, Aristotle discovered in touch an especially intriguing quality that is quite different from all the other senses. Whereas vision is concerned with colors, hearing with sounds, smell with fragrances, the objects of taste and touch do not fall into such easily differentiated categories. Touch, proposed Aristotle, seems to allow us to make accurate assessments of hot and cold, dry and moist, hard and soft, heavy and light, viscous and brittle, rough and smooth, coarse and fine—a succession of intelligent and true contrasts of texture, temperature, and motion. And in this respect touch seems to coincide with taste. Both senses involve "contact," that is, between the organ and the matter from which the pertinent sensation is extracted. Yet, deprived of any knowledge of the workings of the central nervous system, Aristotle had great difficulty in locating the organ with which to connect the sense of touch, unlike vision (eyes), hearing (ears), smell (nose), and taste (tongue). Touch seemed to him to involve far more than merely contact with the skin, as for example when you sense the weight and impact of a heavy object colliding with the shield you hold in your hand, or a tremor in the earth, or the warmth of the sun. The originating agent has not touched you at all, yet you can make an accurate "sense estimate" of hardness, weight, degree of instability, or hotness.

In the end, Aristotle opted for the heart as the most promising seat of the sense of touch, and was strangely disinclined to discover what modern medicine understands well, namely that in our skin and perhaps above all beneath the whorls that cover our fingerpads are concentrated colossally numerous and sensitive nerve endings that moreover enable our brains to monitor the world around us by processing not just one sort of sensory stimulus, but many. What we feel with the fingers of each hand,

and the rest of our skin, is the result of a mind-boggling synthesis and synesthesia. Given his interest in the extremities of other animals—feelers, antennae, the pincers of crabs, the trunks of elephants (an organ of touch *and* smell, but then so is the nose), it seems strange that Aristotle never quite managed to put his finger on touch.

Naturally, in this context, *putting your finger on something* does not only mean to alight upon a correct understanding or to grasp the essence of the matter. In English it also used to mean interfering with it, or, in the case of *laying your finger on someone*, meddling with him or her. Much earlier, *to put the finger in your eye* meant to weep strategically, or to feign weeping, with the worst possible motives. A person suspected of doing this routinely was said to have *a wet finger*.

At least since the phrase first appeared in the Gospel of Matthew (23:4), meanwhile, *not lifting a finger* has meant "to be idle." It is hardly a good thing to be *under someone's thumb*, or to be able *to twist someone around your little finger*, although there are always plenty of people who assume it is. Nor is it clear to me that *having a finger in every pie* is necessarily desirable. *To pull your finger out* is to "get cracking," the implication being that whatever the finger was doing beforehand was at the very least causing delay, presumably the same sense in which, from about 1935, lazy officers of the Royal Air Force were described as having *finger trouble*. In army circles the expression *having your finger well in* conveyed exactly the same meaning.

In criminal slang *to put the finger on someone* meant to inform against that person, while *getting your fingers burned* or *scorched* (that is, snuffing out another man's candle) or *caught in the till* was not usually the result of an accident. In the latter instance, if you were known to have developed the habit of stealing, you were said to be *light-fingered* or, earlier on, to have *fingers made of lime twigs*, or it was said that *each finger was a fish hook*. Nor is *letting something slip through your fingers* in any sense to be envied, except when the context implies an overriding sense of relief or resignation, which is comparatively rare. *Getting your fingers inked* implies carelessness, while *finger-wagging* and *finger-pointing* imply scolding and accusation, maybe groundless. Finally, *giving somebody the finger*, what the French call *"le doigt sale"* (the dirty finger), is obviously now self-explanatory, and belongs with a whole spread of similarly low, formerly exciting senses to which we will return later, including *a bit for the finger*, which once simply meant "woman," and has fortunately now vanished into the upper atmosphere of well-deserved obsolescence.

This point about the strangely distasteful uses to which fingers have been put in English is even clearer when you glance at the uses of *finger* as a verb meaning "to touch with the finger or fingers." This can imply restlessness, unworthy motives, dishonesty, improper desire, even lasciviousness, and betrayal. It can mean to hanker after, to grope, to pilfer, or to cheat. A *fingerer* is not someone you wish to spend a lot of time with. Something that has been *fingered*, then abandoned, is somehow left with a residue of uncleanness, actual or virtual. This also applies to a book that has been *well-thumbed*, though in that event these days one is cheered slightly by the fact that it has been read at all. *Fingering* chess pieces before making a move was in the nineteenth century thought improper.

Although *finger-and-thumb* has a distinguished provenance, having once meant "inseparable," or "forming a superb duo," eventually that admirable sense gave way to cockney slang for *rum*, or *chum* (meaning "companion" or "mate"), and even in various places came to mean "an eccentric or amusing person," in this instance a "low" Australianism, apparently via the poet C. J. Dennis. In the criminal underworld, *finger-and-thumb* was used as an undiluted "term of contempt" for a man or woman, and a *finger's end* eventually came to refer to a racketeer's cut of exactly 10 percent. In the same penumbral society, *finger* was used on its own as a derogatory term explicitly reserved for midwives, policemen, informers, inside men, and pickpockets. Meanwhile, it is not hard to see why few lowly officials appreciate being called a *busmen's finger*; indeed, the lowlier you were, no doubt the more irritating it was.

In fact, for every ten pejorative uses of finger terminology there is scarcely a positive one, and a good proportion of those are steadily vanishing. A *fingerpost* used to mean a road sign, and by association a clergyman, because in theory he pointed the way to Heaven. Not surprisingly, toward the end of the eighteenth century, the English language abandoned the idea of the *fingers* of a clock in favor of *hands*, which, while less logical, were at least free of some of the less attractive senses of finger. (Russian clocks still have fingers.)

The purpose of this book is not to provide an exhaustive history of finger words, or of numbers to the power of ten, hand and finger gestures, or sign languages, or to account for "the finger of scorn," or to trace the complicated development of finger bowls. But in the manner of a trusty coastal lighthouse, it is intended to cast a revolving beam across a surprisingly complicated fingerscape, the particularities of which should make possible further navigation. Clearly there is much here about the representation of fingers in art, and the decoration of real fingers, and ample grounds for suggesting national or cultural tendencies in each case. I think these are powerfully evident. Surely one can trace, for example, a taste in Buddhist sculpture for sinuously curving fingers, a gentle resistance to the whole notion of joint articulation possibly arising from conventions of dance, of delicate motions, as much as one can point to a whole-of-life interest on the part of German and Austrian painters in the expressive potential of long, bony fingers, or sunken phalanges, or swollen joints, and creeping, protruding veins.

French art, meanwhile, exhibits what seems to me an undeniable taste for tiny, not to say minuscule fingertips, and winningly dimpled knuckles. Softness, delicacy, and an impressively independent, free-ranging cocked little finger seem to characterize the digit in French art. There are notable exceptions, above all Antoine Watteau, whose fingers, especially those of string players, tend to be tough, angular, nervy, busily pinning catgut to fretboard, for example, and discovering there delightful chords suitable for Cythera—but the wider trend in French fingers seems to me at least worth considering.

So, too, is the Spanish taste for daringly elongated, narrow fingernails, so readily apparent in the art of El Greco, Velázquez, and Zurbarán, worn as long as the nails of stubbier, far blunter Dutch and Flemish fingers are carefully clipped short; to say nothing of Anthony van Dyck's astonishing way with gloves; or the Victorian obsession with "filbert" nails, or the titanic mid-twentieth-century struggle between the declining glove trade and the new and prospering nail polish business—a phenomenon that, as regards finger imagery, became progressively more and more disengaged from the main currents of fine art, other than high-end fashion, textile design, and maybe cinema.

Even in the work of as great and unconventional a modern master as Pablo Picasso the finger evidently offered enormous expressive potential. There is little that has not already been written, sometimes many times over, about Picasso's *Guernica*, but I have found it surprising how little real attention has been paid to what seems to me the central part played in this political masterpiece by carefully drawn fingers. In all the principal figures—from left to right: the howling mother and child; the prone figure in the foreground; the woman in the window who with outstretched hand clutches the lamp; the seminaked, barefoot woman lunging forward from the right; and the screaming figure behind her, arms raised—the forms of their carefully

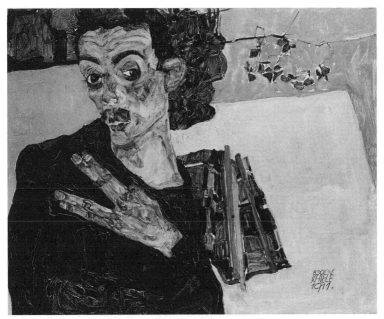

Pushing against the natural restraint imposed by the ligaments that pass across the third and fourth metacarpals, the gesture in Egon Schiele's self-portrait would be neurotic even without his especially nervous handling of bony knuckles and finger joints.

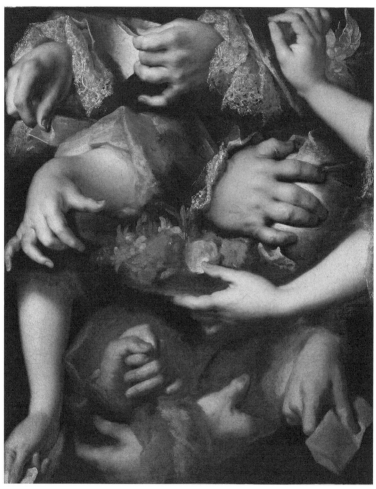

Plump fingers that taper winningly seem to have exercised considerable fascination for French painters from Boucher to Ingres and beyond, as has a freewheeling cocked little finger.

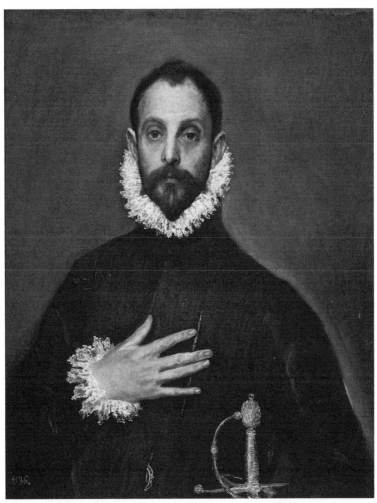

Much reinforced by daringly narrow nails, the elegant fingers of Spanish gentlemen in the portraits of El Greco and Velázquez are as long and attenuated as early Dutch and Flemish fingers are generally short and terminated by the finial of a carefully rounded nail.

sexualized bodies, with armpits and nipples and veins and toe-
nails, are distorted almost to the fullest extent possible without
losing track of what they are doing. But look at all those hands
and stubby fingers, at least twelve sets. With grim determination,
Picasso shows us the limpness of a dead baby's fingers against the
horrifying eloquence of the mother's free hand, the index finger somehow quietly curling toward the thumb in the manner
one occasionally sees in a person overcome by hysteria—creating
in the process an almost perversely correct enumeration of each
set of digits. Fingers clutch, or declaim, or press with long nails
against breasts with sharp nipples. Creased palms and cupped
fingers turn inward, or else thrust outward and upward, the fingers stiffened into swollen lumps that flail or splay or, daringly
enlarged, as in the bottom left-hand corner, simply begin to get
cold. I find it impossible to imagine that in building this great
work of art Picasso was not deeply interested in exploiting the
expressive potential of fingers.

By the period of Picasso's maturity there was a well-established
school of European connoisseurship, specifically in Old Master paintings, which took its lead from Giovanni Morelli,
the nineteenth-century Swiss-Italian scholar and Risorgimento
politician. Morelli attached a great deal of importance to eyes,
ears, fingers, and hands as indicators of an artist's unconscious or
signature style. In simple terms, that line of thinking took as its
starting point the manner in which artists over many hundreds of
years were trained in a busy studio, beginning as apprentices en-
trusted with elementary tasks such as mixing paint and priming
panels and canvases, then gradually building up through careful
instruction and practice a repertoire of increasingly complicated
skills, the culmination of which was the ability to conceive and
execute a complex figure composition on a large scale.

These artist-apprentices usually began the artistic part of their
training by learning many motifs so that they might easily call

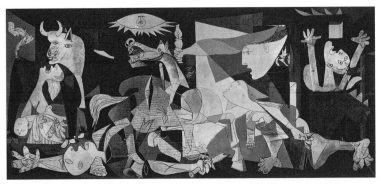

Given the radical structure of his great political masterpiece, the *Guernica* of 1937, Picasso accumulates what seems an almost perversely correct enumeration of each set of digits and each combination of phalanges.

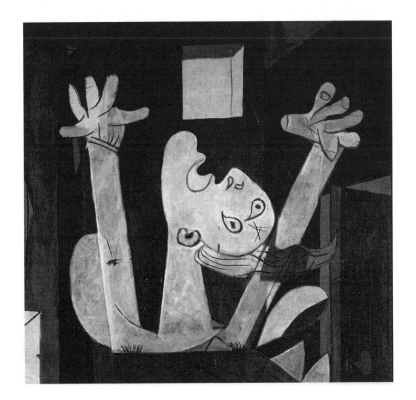

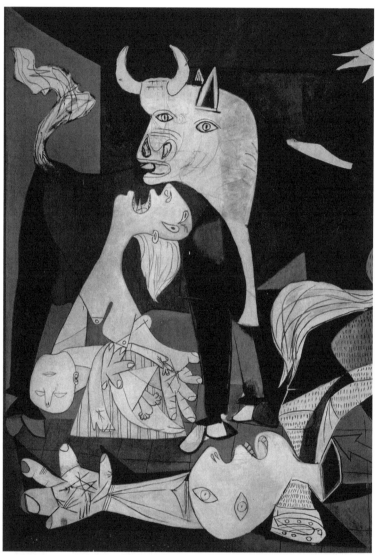

In *Guernica*, each crease separating the finger joints, each wrinkled knuckle and battered terminating nail—a few of them tellingly blackened—is indicated by staccato lines and shapes, chiseled into the composition with slow-burning outrage.

upon them when needed: stones, the folds of draperies, various sorts of foliage, hair, eyes, ears, noses, fingers, and hands. Morelli's insight was that we reveal far more of our true selves through repetitive, rote-learned actions than when we attempt to do something new, big, complicated, or strategic. An independent master with his own studio was less likely to pay particular attention to the deployment in a portrait of, say, the fingers of his sitter's left hand so much as he might give particular thought to the motion or posture of the body, the distinctive shape of the head, the likeness of the face, the delineation of the cheeks and chin and mouth, all of which obviously bore more readily on the function of the portrait than the close observation of actual fingertips. But grasping the bottom rung of this ladder of aesthetic concerns, said Morelli, allows us to point with precision to what eventually, in our era, would become known as the subconscious or unwitting aspect of that master's personal style. In this way you could tell the difference between the work of a master and that of a pupil, or distinguish upon clear grounds between two pictures that in general outline and composition and handling of paint closely resembled each other, but which revealed sharp differences in the handling of lesser, even apparently unimportant motifs such as ears and fingers.

The relatively brief tradition of Morellian connoisseurship powerfully influenced the study of the history of art in the late nineteenth and twentieth centuries. While, inevitably, there must be in any book about fingers a degree of "Morellian" preoccupation, it is neither my intention to drag the reader kicking and screaming through the fingers of Anthony van Dyck or Sir Thomas Lawrence or Pablo Picasso, nor indeed to suggest that such an exercise is especially fruitful apart from helping specialists to reach a consensus as to whether such-and-such an otherwise undocumented picture belongs to Van Dyck's second Antwerp period or his second English period—the fingers of his

English sitters in the court circle of King Charles I are slenderer, and more elegant—or, in the absence of any helpful technical data, whether this Picasso or that Van Gogh is the real thing, or a fake.

I mention Morelli here only because to some extent he helps to explain why, taking as its starting point a few great masterpieces of Western art, a book devoted to the larger subject of fingers, finger imagery, and finger lore has come to be for me more than an arbitrary or even, I daresay, a trivial preoccupation. No doubt there are many philosophical, sociological, cultural, and historical matters arising from the fingers that are only briefly touched on here, and plenty more that others are better qualified than I to tackle. I am not a philosopher. And beyond some reflections on the representation of fingers in art, it is impossible in a relatively short span to do more than select from a limited number of especially intriguing subtopics, such as, for example, the systems of sign language that exist for the benefit of deaf people or Benedictine and Cistercian monks among others, or certain ancient and surprisingly sophisticated systems of finger-based mathematical computation.

The treatment of finger rings, gloves, and nail polish is also necessarily brief, as is the anatomy of the fingers and the hand, with which I commence the next chapter, as well as one miraculous, tiny aspect of DNA that mostly insures, thanks to the so-called Hox genes, that in utero we are hardwired to develop only five of each, and not more, which ought to make better evolutionary sense, if only for the benefit of weavers, harpists, typists, erotomaniacs, and interpreters of the keyboard music of Franz Liszt—evidently Liszt had an exceedingly long ring finger on his right hand.

Above all, this book offers not a Casaubon-like map-and-compass for the human digit, so much as a means by which the finger may point with some precision to curious, often funny, and ever more surprising aspects of us. In writing it, this has been my rule of thumb.

TWO

The Finger and the Hand

What doe we with our hands? Doe we not sue and entreat, promise and performe, call men unto us and discharge them, bid them farewell and be gone, threaten, pray, beseech, deny, refuse, demand, admire, number, confesse, repent, feare, bee ashamed, doubt, instruct, command, incite, encourage, sweare, witnesse, accuse, condemne, absolve, injurie, despise, defie, despight, flatter, applaud, blesse, humble, mocke, reconcile, recommend, exalt, shew gladnesse, rejoyce, complaine, waile, sorrow, discomfort, dispaire, cry out, forbid, declare silence and astonishment: and what not? with so great variation and amplifying as if they would contend with the tongue.

—Michel de Montaigne, *Essays*, Book II, chapter xii, 1580

So complex and intricate is the astonishing mechanism of the hand that for our purposes there is space here only to sketch a few of its basic features, and it is impossible to do so without using anatomical terms, of which *proximal* (nearer, relatively, to the heart) and *distal* (because farther distant) are the most important. The bones of the hand are twenty-seven in number, and project from the distal extremities of the two bones in each forearm, the larger radius, and the slenderer ulna. This is the simplest thing that can be said about them, apart from the fact that the back of the hand is known as the dorsal, and, as luck would have it, the other side is the palmar.

Now, this distinction is both helpful and misleading. It is helpful because each phalanx, or finger bone (plural *phalanges*)— two for the thumb, and three for each of the remaining fingers—and the five metacarpals that underlie the palm and back of the hand and the fleshy base of the thumb, together with their associated muscles, tendons, and many of their motions, conform to the general orientation of front and back. However, that cozy idea entirely fails to describe the remarkably sophisticated "packaging" of the bones of the wrist, the eight carpals (known collectively as the carpus) upon which everything farther distal is utterly dependent.

The inestimable Dr. Henry Gray—a titan of nineteenth-century English medicine who, had he lived beyond the age of thirty-four, would have accumulated many honors, and surely a peerage—arranged the carpal bones into two "rows" of four, which is to me also slightly misleading because the manner in which each of the eight fits snugly next to, and in one instance as many as *seven*, neighboring bones, and up to as many as four of the other carpals could hardly be described as "rowlike." Likewise, hinge, socket, bracket, frame, and ball-bearing metaphors are completely inadequate to describe their amazing interrelationships, but let us not be deflected.

The four proximal bones of the carpus, that is to say, the ones closest to the end of the forearm, consist of (running from thumb side to little finger side) the scaphoid, because it is roughly boat-shaped; the lunate, meaning "moon-shaped"; the triquetrum or triquetral, which is roughly wedgelike; and the pisiform, which nicely resembles half a pea. They form a very approximate crescent sequence, and may be said to "articulate" the wrist and the arm. The first piece of internal logic one should note here is that only the scaphoid and the lunate articulate with the radius, the triquetrum (fitting nicely next to the lunate) being in effect "glued" to the ulna by tough intervening cartilage. We will come to cartilage and ligaments presently, a sticky area.

Upon the relationship between these three carpal bones and the radius and ulna, which may cross each other in the forearm, we therefore depend for our ability to swivel and rotate the wrist, to turn the hand, and to multiply almost infinitely the positions occupied or motions traced by the fingers in three-dimensional space. If you explore the palmar side of your left wrist with the fingers of your right hand (or vice versa), you will feel the big scaphoid projecting somewhat on the thumb side, and the elegant little pisiform sitting patiently against the triquetrum on the little finger side. You may even be able to move it a little from side to side, but be sure to do this gently, as its feelings can easily be hurt.

Just as the upper row of carpals leads from the grand avenue of the forearm into the forecourt knot-garden of the wrist, the lower row of carpals serves to bring about the miraculous transition from that beautiful wrist to the elegant baroque palace of the hand. In other words, the distal carpals provide a springboard for the logically named metacarpals, and thence the phalanges. It is here that the searcher for fingers should be starting to see a glimmer of light. Taken in the same order (from thumb side to little finger side), the lower carpals begin with the irregularly shaped trapezium and the trapezoid, both neatly derived from the Greek word for table, though neither bone looks remotely like a piece of furniture, and one senses that poor Dr. Gray and his earnest predecessors were by this point running out of ideas.

It is on the trapezium that the base of the first metacarpal hinges, and ultimately upon that unique motion, farther down the track, the thumb relies for its ability to "oppose." The trapezoid, meanwhile, is alone among the carpals in supporting the base of only one metacarpal bone, the second and often the longest, the head of which supports the index finger. There is some irony in this, because the trapezoid is the second-to-smallest carpal. Next comes the capitate, so called because it is the largest carpal, forming a sort of hub at the center of the wrist; and, finally, the hamate or unciform, meaning "hooklike." Between them these last two little carpals share the job of supporting the bases of the third, fourth, and fifth metacarpals. Obviously, the range of independent motion that is available to the eight bones of the wrist is extremely restricted; however, it should be emphasized that none of us could perform any manual task more than merely adequately or even at all if we lacked a single one.

While the metacarpals are the anatomical basement story of the fingers, and the first of them is considerably more than that—in so many ways the Napoleon of the family, far shorter, stouter, more versatile, and inventively mobile than its siblings—it should not be forgotten that the bases of the remaining four metacarpals do more than merely sit meekly against the relevant carpals, looking chic. They afford considerable strength and flexibility to the hand by articulating with one another as well, the second with the third, the third with the second and fourth, and the fourth with the third and fifth. This interdependence makes possible the cupping or squeezing into a surprisingly narrow circumference the "flat" of the hand, having to some degree the restricted but at the same time surprisingly variable range of motion that you can observe when you clutch the bases of five pencils between your thumb and index finger and, allowing them to radiate or flare a little, with the other hand you test the mobility of each at the other, free end.

Somewhat surprisingly, the second through fifth metacarpals may often descend gradually in length, and do not always correspond with the relative dimensions of the fingers that spring from them. The metacarpals are also slightly slenderer than the phalanges in the fingers because, being held in relatively tight discipline between the palm and the back of the hand, they gain strength in numbers and in any case are not required to function nearly as independently as the freewheeling digits. Thus Dr. Gray's phrase "they are long, cylindrical bones presenting for examination a shaft and two extremities" seems dry, and somewhat ungenerous. If the phalanges are the elite shock troops, to shift metaphors again, advancing daringly ahead of the other bones of the hand, and the carpals, meanwhile, are its staff officers in closed conference at the rear, the metacarpals, it seems to me, are its corps of engineers—dependable, in fact indispensable, but often given insufficient credit for their quiet strength and ingenuity.

When we run the tips of the fingers of one hand across the knuckles of the other, it is not the base of the proximal phalanx of each finger that we are feeling underneath the tendons—we shall get to those presently—so much as the bigger, stronger head of the corresponding metacarpal. You can also feel between your knuckles how much more freedom of movement (free, that is, from each other) the last four metacarpals attain at the head than is permitted at the tight conjunction of their bases, though of course the structure and interrelationship of the metacarpals has necessarily evolved to provide brilliantly both for strength *and* flexibility. They are miniature masterpieces.

Our fingers consist of fourteen separate phalanges. The proximal phalanges are the ones that finger rings mostly surround. The "lowest," corresponding with the fingertips, are called the distal phalanges; the remainder, of course, forming a middle row (except for the thumb). In fact, the thumb lacks a middle phalanx partly because its metacarpal operates rather like a phalanx, and if you fold your thumb right across the palm of your hand and touch with its tip the fleshy mound (known as the hypothenar eminence) immediately distal to the proximal phalanx of your little finger, you will see that for this reason an additional, middle or third phalanx in the thumb is hardly necessary, and would no doubt strike us as unattractive except to infants and people who harbor an eccentric desire to touch their wrist with the thumbtip of the same hand.

Now, all of the joints that separate the twenty-seven bones

of the hand, and many other joints in the human body, are of course movable, and the anatomical term for these is *synovial*. Some joints are of course thankfully immovable, such as the ones in the skull and pelvis. The ends of the bones that meet in synovial joints are coated with slippery, smooth articular cartilage, which prevents them from scraping unpleasantly against each other when we set them in motion, rattling indiscreetly, or wearing out too soon. With age, or as a result of injury, cartilage can be torn or damaged or simply worn away, causing pain, and articular cartilage is no different. However, what holds two bones together at these joints, ideally allowing them to move freely but tightly against each other within orderly limits, is the ligaments. In most cases, the movement of the bones is further lubricated by means of a tiny cushion of synovial fluid, which is produced by a group of cells servicing each joint that is called the synovium, and that fluid is contained within a, yes, synovial membrane, which the ligaments enclose, or at least ideally prevent getting squashed out of position.

The ligaments consist of bands of mostly white fibrous tissue, extraordinarily dense, tight, pliant, strong, elastic, and resilient. If it were simply the case that ligaments crossed from bone to proximate bone, their importance to the structure and the motion of the hand would be a good deal easier to explain—and the hand itself rather floppy, comparatively useless, and frankly depressing. However, as well as providing the little Japanese bridges between individual bones and parts of bones (à la Claude Monet), the ligaments, especially those of the carpal or wrist joints (anterior and posterior, that is, front and back), and certain amazing ligament-forming membranes and sheets of cartilage, not all of them taut, form a veritable Los Angeles "four-level interchange," an Orange Crush of multilayered, multidirectional overpasses and connectors, the purpose of which is to allow the degree of flexibility we have in our hands, while at the same time making the bones and range of motions as secure and predictable as they possibly can be.

Stretchy ligaments hold bones together at the joints, but what set them in motion are the muscles and the tendons, which likewise in various forms go from bone to bone, or in many cases from other muscles to bone, or merge to form bigger, stronger tendons, one end of which is normally anchored to a bone. In some respects tendons also resemble ligaments in that they are essentially strong, white, fibrous cords, and can also take many different forms—rounded, flat, razor thin, or impressively thick (as in the sturdy Achilles)—and extend from short to long distances depending on their role. On the other hand (and in almost any other context I would not need to underline the fact that here, dear reader, I speak *figuratively*), tendons are fundamentally different from ligaments because, in the words of Dr. Gray, they are "devoid of elasticity," the better to fulfill their function as anchors on the bones for muscles or certain sets of muscles that taper down to the tendons, and to make sure that when we flex that muscle, the resulting movements of bone-in-joint are exact and immediate. If tendons were as elastic as ligaments, at best the world would be waist-deep in broken china, and freeways would be considerably more dangerous than they already are.

The principal drawback of tendons is that there is very little blood supplied to them, so that when they are damaged or torn—and generations of hearty sportsmen will attest to the fact that it takes an almighty yank to achieve this—it takes them a very long time to heal, and sometimes they can be permanently weakened.

Like the mesh of ligaments in the hand, which for our purposes are too numerous and complicated to list and explain in full, though Dr. Gray achieved this awesome task, the muscles and tendons that manipulate the bones that meet in the joints form one of the most remarkable and intricate spheres of mo-

tor function with which we humans are equipped. This general
point increases ten-, twenty-, even a hundredfold when you take
into account the complexities of the vascular system and those
dozens of branches of the arteries that under relatively enormous, continual pressure from the heart keep the muscles of the
arm, wrist, and hand supplied with rich, red, oxygenated blood;
and the veins, which rather more sluggishly return post hoc blue
blood to cardiac headquarters; to say nothing of the twin roles
of the so-called median, ulnar, and radial nerves, and their many
branches, namely to allow your brain to stimulate those muscles
and flex them, and to receive, process, and respond to a ceaseless supply of, at best, extremely helpful and, at worst, extremely
painful sensory information, all of it in an instant hurrying back
up essentially the same neurological pathways.

The quality of that information is extraordinarily high.
Between them the different kinds of receptors that are stimulated and in turn stimulate the nerve endings embedded in our
skin enable our hands to detect minute quantities of pressure,
changes in temperature, degrees of vibration, and not merely
the presence but also the location, direction, speed, distinctness,
and number of tactile motions across the surface of our skin.
They may let some of us differentiate between real beaver and
synthetic, between rough surfaces and smooth, between a ba-
nana skin and orange peel, between flat and undulating surfaces,
between nearly identical objects of very slightly different size,
between soft and hard. They insure that when, assisted by the
eye, we reach out and pick up a hen's egg—the action known as
prehension—judging both by the degree of friction afforded by
the surface of the eggshell, and the amount of pressure from the
fingertips that is needed to secure the egg, we manage to do so
without breaking or dropping it. There are, of course, limits to
the nuances of sensation available at our fingertips. Depending
on the size of the ant that crawls across our knuckles, there are
quite a lot of us who may hardly detect its presence at all, but

few of us who do feel it would be able to differentiate among each of its six separate footfalls, or the action of its two antennae. Its bite is quite another matter.

Finally, there is the astounding capacity of the outermost organ, the skin, to allow your hands and fingers not merely to stretch and fold, permitting a full range of motion, but to hold every one of these constituent parts, from bone up to knuckle hair and fingernail, more or less in its correct spot. We shall consider fingernails later on. Keep in mind that this is by no means all that the skin does. Perspiration, that simple process which, as well as regulating temperature, expelling dirt, and providing much-needed traction for fingertips active in slippery circles, is merely one of the many other capacities of the skin that on its own constitutes a minor miracle. That the human skin does all this and much else besides, under conditions of incessant, often energetic, sometimes involuntary activity, dramatically fluctuating temperatures, and a Niagara of sensory bombardment, while at the same time managing also, for example, to repair itself and replace almost as new the papillary ridges that form whorls and other patterns which cover the outermost palmar surface of each of your fingertips when from time to time they get nicked or cut—these capacities are, or should be, enough to stimulate rapt meditations on the wonder of creation, and this is not even to scratch the surface, as we shall see.

Every component I have mentioned so far—bones, joints, ligaments, muscles, tendons, blood vessels, nerves, and skin, each of which merits a chapter of its own (I do not propose to go into the lymphatic system, which when it does not work properly can, among other things, cause one limb to grow very much larger than the other, a result of the pathological condition known as lymphedema)—is needed for the fingers and the hand effectively to perform their infinitely variable motions, with the possible exception of knuckle hair, which appears to be a vestigial remnant left behind in the most recent stages of our evo-

lution. Yet it is the sheer range, variety, and intricacy of those
motions, especially any that require the opposition of the thumb,
in which we may discover a simple explanation for why we humans are who we are, and how far these unique capacities have
set us apart from all other mortal creatures, and yielded the inestimable gift of civilization, with all its benefits, responsibilities,
and opportunities for folly and abuse.

We may observe the sheer magnificence of the entire system by applying all that we have considered up to this point to
those two exquisite gestures by which Michelangelo Buonarroti
represented the creation of man in the middle of the ceiling of
the Sistine Chapel in Rome. If one were totally to obliterate the
poetry of that conjunction of the right hand of God the Father
and the left hand of the awakening Adam (the name is ancient
Hebrew for "man"), one might draft the following ashen but I
hope in the present context useful sentences.

In their respectively recumbent positions—God borne
aloft by angels, Adam reclining on the six-day-old earth—let us
imagine that the arms and hands that nearly meet at the center
of the composition have moved from a position of rest into the
alignment in which Michelangelo observed them in his artist's
models. Setting aside for obvious reasons of brevity the astonishing functions of the shoulder and upper body, which require
another book, we can draw a few anatomical conclusions from
what we see: In the forearm of God and that of Adam also, inter
alia, the muscle we call the *pronator teres*, having been supplied
with blood by the radial artery in the forearm, and stimulated by
the muscular branches of the median nerve (among others)—
this vital muscle has evidently been flexed, and the radius and
ulna have been deftly swiveled. The corresponding muscles that
cause the opposite motion, likewise supplied with blood by the
radial artery in the forearm, and also stimulated by the muscular
branches of the median nerve (among others)—these are relaxed.

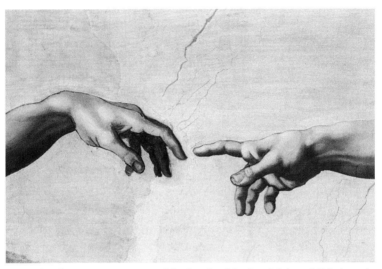

Upon this famous convergence of the hands of God and Adam, Michelangelo imposed an ingenious combination of hints about kindred resemblance and contrasting signs of age.

It is important to observe that these muscles essentially function in tandem, in push-me-pull-you mode, and they constitute merely a crudely selected example of the enormous sum of motions set in train and contained within the muscles of the forearm. These are what orient the wrist of God and the wrist of Adam so that the palmar surface of each is, at least pictorially, downward-facing.

Traveling farther toward the fingertips, we may also observe what we see in the general shape of our own hands every day, namely the powerful muscles of the thumb which together produce the fleshy, so-called thenar eminence—there it is, the cheeky thing, swelling nicely (I hope) between your wrist and the base of your thumb. If it is not, you may wish to seek and follow medical advice. What we cannot see so well, not more than in faint profile, is God's slightly less powerful but immensely important muscles of the little finger—they are the ones that essentially make up the entire little-finger side of your hand, and are with ineffable logic known as the hypothenar eminence. Adam's is completely invisible. This is because here, in Michelangelo, it has ended up positioned on the far side of his left hand, and is therefore obscured from view.

Now, God has not merely set in train the whole act of creation, but among the many other muscles of His hand, He is also here evidently flexing the muscle in His forearm that is called the *extensor indicis*, but not its near neighbors the *extensors digitorum* or *digiti minimi*—which is how God's index finger comes to be extended yet the phalanges ever so slightly curved or flexed, producing that beautiful line; while the middle, ring, and little fingers are relaxed, with only the slightest hint of flexion in the little finger, over the middle joint of which the artist has plotted the exquisitely observed shadow of God's thumb. The same observations are to some extent also true of Adam's hand, although the contractions of the same muscles are in every case fainter, as befits the subject: man awakening for the first time. Meanwhile, God's thumb is extending; that is to say, his *extensors pollicis longus* and *pollicis brevis*, and to a lesser extent the *abductor pollicis*, are all at work, while Adam's are apparently not.

This exercise might be carried forward in limitlessly tedious detail; however, the point I am making so bluntly is that what Michelangelo here achieves by means of careful observation and artistic synthesis conveys also the internal logic that both governs the mechanisms and functions of our hands, and equips them with the enormous range of uses and capacities for nonverbal expression that each of us exploits continually. One final observation serves to nudge this scale of considerations back toward the artist himself.

With the brilliance of a poet and painter of rarely equaled capacities, Michelangelo brings to his orchestration of these two marvelous hands several daring but anatomically cogent points of interpretation. The hands of God and Adam are alike. They carry a family resemblance. The profile of the index fingers is that of father and son. The middle and ring fingers, meanwhile, rest against each other, reflecting not merely the relatively constraining effect of those muscles, tendons, and ligaments whose natural restrictions cause them to do this naturally, but offering at the same time a further, powerfully suggestive hint of likeness. Yet Michelangelo has carefully inscribed each hand with contrasting signs of age. The joints of God's thumb are bigger and maybe stronger; the nail is broader, perhaps worn, even pared, at any rate squared off. This is a tougher, older hand. The fingertips are slightly blunter. Those two powerful hand-manipulating tendons of the muscles of the forearm that are known as the *palmaris longus* and the *flexor carpi radialis*—flex your wrist and there you can see them for yourself, on the palmar side: up they come—God's are bigger and more prominent, and are shown protruding much farther up His forearm than Adam's. Meanwhile, the squashy slackness of the skin over the last interphalangeal joint of God's thumb—skin that, with dismay, you will see for yourself gets squashier and wrinklier with each passing year, and if you are too young to observe this now we shall have this conversation again in five or ten years' time—finds an eloquent response in the smooth thumb joint of Adam. Indeed, all these qualities in the digit, hand, and wrist of God are contrasted point for point by the slenderness, smoothness, and relaxation of the hand and wrist of Adam, even down to his tender, ovoid thumbnail. It is tempting to speculate whether in painting these hands at close quarters against those days' portions of the ceiling fresco, Michelangelo indulged in the vanity of carrying into the divine hand something of the strength and maturity of his own, and inscribing on Adam's the beautiful shapes and contours he admired in a much younger hand, possibly mixing paint and washing brushes nearby.

As anyone who suffers from rheumatoid arthritis will gladly attest (more women than men, alas), there is much that can go wrong with hands. The list of ailments and pathologies is as long as your arm. Precisely because the fingers range so freely in space, touching, grasping, tapping, poking, and prodding—incessant corporeal busybodies—before the advent of the motor car they were obviously at greater risk of physical injury than something as formidably protected as your kidneys, spleen, or pancreas. Moreover, history teaches that until very recently what we now regard as trivial ailments, cuts, even pinpricks to healthy fingers or thumbs often resulted in serious infections, sometimes gangrene, and regularly caused death after usually long and agonizing illnesses.

That fascinating catalog of horrors the criminal *Proceedings of the Old Bailey* yields a number of late-seventeenth-century trials for murder arising from gangrenous wounds to the finger that in the space of sometimes only a month caused the death of the victim. In every case, the defendants were acquitted not because of what we would today regard as the relatively slight nature of the wound, but instead because it could not be proven that any of them had cut the finger and therefore committed the crime, or that the digital misadventure had not been an accident. In July 1682, a jury acquitted one "Edling" of the murder of a Mr. Stanley, who, treated by "several Chyrurgeons," survived for an agonizing two years and three months after his finger was nicked in a scuffle in Westminster Abbey Yard, during which time first his finger, then his hand, and finally his whole arm was successively amputated, obviously without success.

By the end of the eighteenth century, the prospects of people with damaged fingers were beginning to improve, although today we tend to read as quaint or trivial a relatively long newspaper report about the actress and singer Mrs. Billington having had to cancel a London appearance in *Robin-Hood* because of soreness arising from a pinprick to her thumb, an accident sustained while sewing a yellow chin-stay to her husband's nightcap. *The Times* noted that the swelling had dampened the spirit of her singing "not a little," but that a surgeon was attending. Lady Maria Wentworth, a daughter of Lord Cleveland, was not so fortunate when, at the end of the sixteenth century, she died "in consequence of pricking her finger with a needle, while making up child-bed linen for the poor." From Scotland in January 1802 reliable intelligence to the effect that the Duke of Queensberry had been attacked by gout in his little finger was evidently considered newsworthy, and serious.

Even as lately as the 1860s and 1870s, the English law columns regularly reported on extremely high sums sought from rich and powerful railway companies on the grounds of negligence for injuries to digits, as in two nearly identical cases in which a passenger's thumb was crushed in a compartment door when an overenthusiastic porter slammed it shut. In 1866, at the Guildford assizes, Mr. Justice Willes found in favor of the plaintiff, Mr. Simmons, a "fancy box-maker" of London, who was thus injured on the Metropolitan line at Farringdon Street. The other case, fought vigorously for more than six years and cunningly referred to by counsel on behalf of the Metropolitan Railway Company as the "pinched thumb case," eventually in 1877 reached the Judicial Committee of the Privy Council, on appeal. At length their lordships decided to reverse the decision of several lower courts to award costs amounting to more than two thousand pounds, and damages. Both cases make Dickens's Jarndyce and Jarndyce seem open and shut. In other words, modern medicine and reconstructive surgery have prevailed against numerous terrible illnesses for which our digits once offered a convenient and devastating foothold.

Yet apart from accidentally crushed or even lopped digits, numerous ailments may arise from the compression of nerves in the arm and hand, or from acute inflammatory conditions that, like cuts on the hand or fingers, were far more serious before the arrival of antibiotics, to say nothing of the many different kinds of swelling or lesion that can overcome any kind of tissue in the hand anywhere from the bedrock of bone up to the surface of the skin. And this is not even to consider congenital conditions.

We shall return to certain physical aspects of the finger and the hand as we go along, but in conclusion it is worth mentioning what is for me perhaps the most astonishing thing of all. Since the titanic achievement of decoding the human genome was completed not so long ago, we now know that the genes responsible for regulating the development or morphogenesis of practically all living things are the subset known as the homeobox. Of these, a subgroup known as the Hox genes are responsible for among other things determining the location of limbs, and the development in utero of discrete arrangements of bones, organs, blood vessels, skin, and so on—bringing order to the awesome multiplication of millions upon millions of living cells, each and every one of which contains the genetic blueprint that ensures they are what they should be, and will eventually do what they are supposed to do. As our bodies take shape in the womb, a further subset of Hox genes—that, incidentally, we share with many species, including, somewhat surprisingly, sponges, starfish (obviously), bats, and chickens—ensure that we develop from the tiny "limb bud" no more and no fewer than five fingers on each hand and five toes on each foot. The determining influence of the Hox genes on the manner in which the hand develops in utero is total, and in those cases when the glitch or mutation of polydactyly occurs, and we leap from the womb with an extra digit, that finger is in fact merely a replica or accidental duplicate of one of the canonical five, often severely limited in motion and usefulness, and not a freewheeling or independently grown sixth. This distinction is vital.

It was once thought that almost alone among the mammals, the panda was inexplicably equipped with a sixth, thumblike digit with which it takes hold of bamboo for ease of nibbling. However, that anomalous extremity, it now turns out, is not a digit at all but an enormously extended or lengthened bone in the panda's wrist (the radial sesamoid) that, in evolutionary terms, took a long detour and has consequently acquired a certain amount of mobility and usefulness, but is strictly speaking not a digit. So the "rule of five" applies even to our panda cousins.

For reasons that need not get in our way just now, a related subgroup of Hox genes is also closely involved with the development of the sex organs of both men and women. No doubt this will raise the question at the back of the classroom as to why men do not develop an exciting array of five penises and women five clitorises. The answer would appear to be that to set in train the further miracle of human reproduction only one of each is ever necessary and, while no doubt amusing, any more than that would be an indulgence and occasionally inconvenient.

What is so curious about the Hox genes and their determining role is that the "rule of five" is somewhat counterintuitive, because it ought to have made better evolutionary sense for species to acquire advantage over the millennia from an increasing number of digits, to cast the net of sensory perception even wider, to accomplish any number of complex tasks with greater dispatch. For some reason, perhaps relating to the fundamental place in the genome that is occupied by any genes that determine morphogenesis—because if these begin to change in unstable or comparatively unpredictable directions, then there is nothing but chaos all the way down the developmental line—or else to the operation of some innate principle equivalent to that of diminishing returns, the rule of five has proven rock solid, at least in evolutionary biological terms. Will seven fingers on each hand let me hang on to the branch of a tree, extract a gull's egg from the nest, or throw a stone at my enemy any more effectively than five? Ichthyologists know that the anal fin of certain male fish in the families of Anablepidae and Poeciliidae does not seem to have benefited from a greater number of spines than five, although with hair-raising inventiveness the third, fourth, and fifth have modified themselves to form a movable thing called a *gonopodium*, with which the males like to impregnate the females. In other words, small evolutionary marvels have occurred, but they occur while observing this fundamental rule of five. Indeed, as Neil Shubin has lately pointed out, the evolutionary scheme of many limbs of many creatures seems to have developed in remarkable conformity to the shared or common plan of one bone, followed by two bones, followed by a collection of small, bloblike bones, then five digits—this is as true of the extinct theropod dinosaur, the extinct pterosaur, the claw of the lizard, the foot of the chicken, the flipper of the seal, and the wing of the bat as it is true of the extremities of *Homo sapiens*. Indeed, the bat has never flapped better or farther by accumulating more than the five distal bones that have lately supported each wing (even though one of these, the "thumb," sprouting from the "elbow," seems at first glance oddly superfluous). In assuming their vital role in bat propulsion, those five bones gradually recombined and elongated themselves in a manner little short of dazzling; however, they have never shown any inclination to add to their number, nor retrench. They are five, and will remain so for as long as bats flap rowdily and defecate all over the Royal Botanic Gardens in Melbourne.

Above all, while they have obviously evolved in shape, length, maneuverability, and disposition—to our ultimate benefit—the digits of the higher primates, fingers and toes, have always conformed to the same predictable pattern of number, and despite the regular occurrence of the late mutations that cause polydactyly and syndactyly, the entire mechanism of the human hand has emerged and triumphed under the higher jurisdiction of the strict court of Hox, from which there is thankfully no appeal.

THREE

The Finger of God

And he gave unto Moses, when he had made an end of communing
with him upon Mount Sinai, two tables of testimony, tables of stone,
written with the finger of God.   —Book of Exodus, 31:18

I can count on the fingers of one hand the number of aesthetic
experiences that one would willingly call life-changing—and
I have a full set of fingers. One of these occurred some years ago,
on a visit to the great thirteenth-century temple in Kyoto called
the Rengeōin or, more popularly, the Sanjūsangendō, which
means "Temple of the Thirty-three Bays." This enormous, plain,
shoebox-shaped wooden building houses a colossal statue of
Kannon, the feminine manifestation of Avalokiteśvara, the bodhisattva of infinite compassion. She sprouts forty-two arms, and
a forest of hands. An eleven-foot-high masterpiece of Japanese
sculpture of the Kamakura period (1185–1333 C.E.), Kannon is
gloriously flanked by her heavenly cosmic guardians or attendants,
the twenty-eight so-called *bushū*, and one thousand life-sized,
eleven-headed, "thousand-armed" standing statues, representing
different versions of herself, carved in cypress wood, then gilded.
Each statue is carefully differentiated from the next and, like its
larger prototype, has dozens of pairs of hands, the fingers painstakingly crafted into a bewildering range of delicate gestures.

These statues fill the temple, and are carefully accommodated on a gigantic altar consisting of ten ascending steps that accommodate these seemingly numberless ranks of statues. It is said that all Japanese pilgrims should be able to discover their own face peering back from this host of silent bodhisattvas, who, like them, await a higher incarnation. Their fingers are exquisite.

The religious instinct, which is as old as man, and has in many quarters come in for harsh criticism lately, has often displayed a formidable tendency to conceive and worship an anthropomorphic divinity in whose image mankind was made, or a pantheon of divinities in whom the full range of human strengths and weaknesses could be seen to originate. With the notable exception of Islam, which specifically renounces the concept of an anthropomorphic godhead, this seems to be one of the things that the ancient world religions have in common. And, as Albert E. Elsen once remarked, the history of art amply demonstrates that in responding to this idea, evidently we humans have continually sought in God, and gods, powerfully charismatic images of ourselves.

Where it existed and still exists, centuries of theological speculation have periodically but continually refined this basic, anthropomorphic pattern, so that in the early centuries of Christianity, for example, the concept rapidly solidified of a triune deity consisting of the painstakingly differentiated but mystically indivisible Father, Son, and Holy Spirit. It is no accident that in the developing conventions of the primitive church various gestures of benediction attributed to Jesus himself, and also dispensed by priests and bishops, assumed three principal forms: (a) the thumb, index, and middle fingers of the right hand are extended, and the ring and little fingers of the same hand folded over; occasionally the thumb is brought over and tucked into the furrow separating the index and middle fingers; (b) the tip of the ring finger touches the tip of the thumb, while the in-

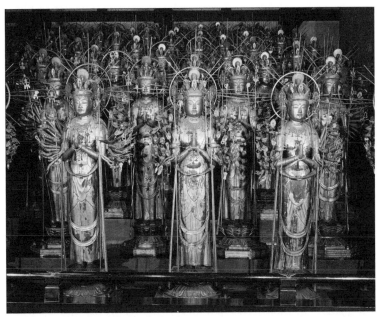

The Sanjūsangendō in Kyoto, Japan, was built to accommodate one thousand of these dazzling gilded personifications of Avalokiteśvara, the bodhisattva of infinite compassion, as well as a much larger seated parent statue and twenty-eight bushū, or warrior-guardians.

dex, middle, and little fingers are extended; and (c) the index and little fingers are extended, while the tips of the middle and ring fingers touch the tip of the thumb. In whichever of these three different positions, the hand so configured traces the sign of the cross. And in the hieratic imagery of the Eastern Empire these precise conventions or attitudes of benediction were with equal if not greater power and formality impressed upon most subsequent images in mosaic and sculpture of Christ the Priest King. The theology of icons, over which in the eighth century a long and acrimonious civil war was fought and ultimately won, conceived of images of God as an exposition of the doctrine of the incarnation—God assumed human form in Jesus, and that the members of the Trinity may each be represented at all was said to constitute powerful, unarguable evidence of the truth of that proposition. Moreover, the Christ who thus raises His right hand in the gesture of benediction does so, in a sense, from the vantage point of the here and now, seated on the throne of judgment in Heaven, where He reigns and ever shall until He returns in glory at the end of time. In Byzantine terms, these gestures carry a mystic blessing, but they stand as a complex theological analog also, and as a promise. Priests and bishops in many branches of modern Christianity still proffer them, though these days paying rather less attention to the formal disposition of the digits.

Centuries earlier than the arrival of Christianity, the pantheons of ancient Near Eastern, Greek, and Roman religion, and of various branches of Hinduism, similarly worshipped gods in basically human form, occasionally hybrid, but mostly recognizable as exempla of men and women—wiser, craftier, more beautiful, and variously omnipotent. Spreading rapidly from the Indian subcontinent, successive schools of Indian, Himalayan, and, later, Chinese and Japanese Buddhism conceived the various types of bodhisattva—"proto-Buddha," or enlightenment being—including

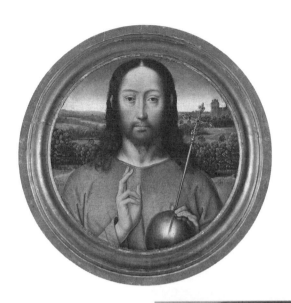

ABOVE: Christ, the "Saviour of the World," adopts a right-handed gesture of benediction in which the thumb and index and middle fingers stand for the members of the Holy Trinity.

RIGHT: In many Byzantine and later icons of Christ Pantocrator (the All-Powerful), the gesture of benediction is composed slightly differently, though the symbolism is the same.

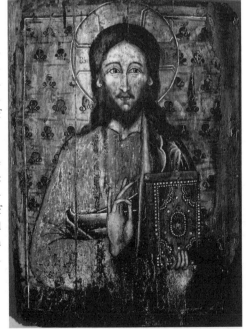

Kannon (who in China is known as Guanyin), and they, too, mostly derive their notional form from the human body.

Within the enormously complex and variegated history of Buddhism there are numerous working definitions of bodhisattva. In the earliest traditions this malleable concept referred exclusively to the degrees of enlightenment gradually attained during his lifetime by the one Lord Buddha himself. Before long, however, it came to refer to the aspiration to Buddhahood, and to postulants who, out of compassion, vowed "to become a Buddha for the sake of all sentient beings." Gradually these two divided frameworks of celestial bodhisattva and "bodhisattva practice" were reconciled by carefully enumerating and distinguishing among the stages of development embraced by each—the spiritual growth or enlightenment processes on earth mirroring those in heaven. Bodhisattvas came to be arranged in ascending ranks, but they were far more than milestones on the road to enlightenment. In Mahayana Buddhism, for example, each bodhisattva was said to provide the example of a standardized set of ten stages of enlightenment, which applied both to celestial and earthly practice. This mode of thought was enormously influential, and while much of the original literature in Sanskrit has been lost—it is thought that it ran to hundreds of thousands of verses—some of it survives in rare Tibetan and Chinese translations dating from the Tang period. And it is to these humanoid bodhisattva concepts (and variants) that much of the spiritual and devotional life of Hinduism and Buddhism cleave, never more pertinently in the present context than by developing an enormous body of mudras, to which we shall turn presently.

Other than to their adherents, perhaps, in purely cultural terms the Judeo-Christian traditions present a far more straightforward anthropomorphism than the bodhisattva framework permits, or indeed the huge pantheons of ancient Near Eastern deities. Whereas in Judaism the disembodied voice of God thun-

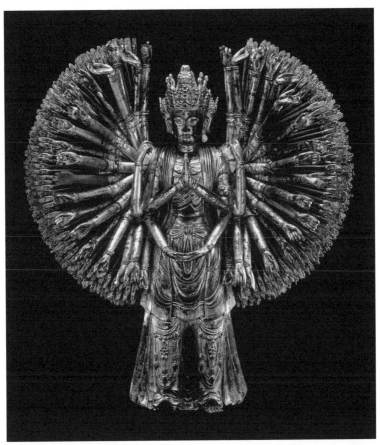

The Chinese variant of Kannon, the feminine manifestation of Avalokiteśvara, the bodhisattva of infinite compassion, is known as Guanyin, and is held to sprout one thousand arms, and therefore five thousand fingers, the foremost of which are made to adopt carefully disposed mudras, or gestures of the fingers and head.

ders back to Moses from the burning bush, "I am who I am"—
words that reverberate so enigmatically, so powerfully from the
exceedingly ancient text of Exodus—elsewhere and often the
Hebrew scriptures are dense with references to a mighty, humanoid king-deity, *YHWH*, who Isaiah says "shall not judge by
what his eyes see, or decide by what his ears hear" but with that
righteousness which "shall be the belt around his waist," according to which, if necessary, "with the breath of his lips he shall
kill the wicked." Here the powerful imagery of eyes, ears, a waist,
and lips is unavoidable; and when Moses ascends Mount Sinai to
receive the stone tablets of the law, they are inscribed with the
very finger of God.

Hands and hand imagery are as commonplace in the Bible
as they are everywhere else. In Genesis alone, God declares that
man must not reach out his hand and pick from the tree of life
(3:22). Angrily, he declares that the earth has received the blood
of Abel from the hand of Cain (4:11). The father of Noah sees
the patriarch as the promise of comfort "concerning our work
and the toil of our hands" (5:29). The same Noah puts forth his
hand from the ark and receives the portentous dove (8:9). After
the flood he is blessed, sent forth to multiply and replenish the
earth: "The fear of you and the dread of you shall be upon every
beast of the earth, and upon every fowl of the air, upon all that
moveth upon the earth, and upon all the fishes of the sea; into
your hand are they delivered" (9:2). In due course the enemies
of Abraham are delivered into his hand (14:20), and two verses
later the patriarch responds by lifting up the same hand to "the
Lord, the most high God." Much later, in chapter 22, the hand
of Abraham assumes vital importance in the extraordinary account of the Sacrifice of Isaac, which Christians came to see
as a vital precursor of the Passion. "Lay not thy hand upon the
lad," says the angel of the Lord, "neither do thou anything unto
him: for now I know that thou fearest God, seeing thou hast

not withheld thy son, thine only son from me." Later still, in his blindness old Isaac fails to distinguish between his sons Jacob and Esau because, according to the text, both have *very* hairy hands (27:22–23).

The whole of Genesis and indeed the Pentateuch are populated by hands of supplication, worship, and work; hands into which divine blessings are delivered, and hands, such as that of Pharaoh, from which in turn the posterity of Abraham and Moses are saved. There are hands that build, hands conjoined in marriage, and hands that yield burnt offerings according to the word of the Lord. One might even conceive of all five books of Moses as a manual for the people of Israel.

And although the hand is omnipresent in Hebrew scripture, discrete fingers are mentioned far less often but quite strategically. In the five books of Moses, they conform to a small number of carefully chosen contexts. In Exodus (8:19), for example, Pharaoh's magicians discern a ghastly plague of gnats as the retributive "finger of *YHWH*," not the hand of God but his finger. Later, Moses receives the stone tablets of the law neatly inscribed with the same divine finger. The Gospel of Luke (11:20) has Jesus employing the same vivid term: "But if it is by *the finger of God* that I cast out demons, then the Kingdom of God has come upon you." It seems likely that within the conventions governing these early scriptures the divine finger was an especially pointed evocation of God's imminence, a declaration of His creative as distinct from His destructive power, and maybe above all His direct involvement in human affairs.

As well, in a narrower sense, elaborate cleansing and anointing rituals of the Israelites carefully stipulate the use of the index finger dipped in the blood of sacrificed animals (Exodus 29:12, Leviticus 4:6, and so on), while later there is the finger-pointing of accusation (Isaiah 58.9), the finger of threat and combat (Job 1:12, Psalm 144:1–2), finger and thumb torture (Judges 1:6–7), as well as the sinister mark of polydactyly—Jonathan slays a Philistine giant with six on each hand (2 Samuel 21:20–21). There is even occasionally the beautiful, even fragrant finger of sensuality (Song of Songs 5:5); the nimble finger of manual dexterity (Proverbs 31:19); and the finger of indolence, that is, not lifting it (Matthew 23:4, Luke 11:46). Most of these finger-related figures of biblical speech are not only exceedingly ancient, but persist healthily in our time.

Elsewhere in the canonical Gospels finger imagery is deployed with breathtaking effectiveness, as in the parable of the rich man and Lazarus when, seeing him resting in the bosom of Abraham, the rich man cries out from Hell: "Have mercy on me, and send Lazarus to dip the end of his finger in water and cool my tongue, for I am in anguish in this flame!" (Luke 16:24). Even more memorably, appearing to the disciples after the Resurrection, Jesus bids Thomas to put *his finger* into the open wound in his side, that he might "stop doubting and believe" (John 20:27). However, one of the most surprising and inexplicable references to the divine finger in the New Testament relates directly to the act of writing, and comes in the episode of the woman taken in adultery, the so-called *pericope adulterae* in the Gospel of John (8:3–11):

> The scribes and the Pharisees brought a woman who had been caught in adultery, and placing her in the midst they said to him, "Teacher, this woman has been caught in the act of adultery. Now in the law Moses commanded us to stone such. What do you say about her?" This they said to test him, that they might have some charge to bring against him. *Jesus bent down and wrote with his finger on the ground.* And as they continued to ask him, *he stood up and said to them,* "Let him who is without sin among you be the first to throw a stone at her." *And once more*

he bent down and wrote with his finger on the ground. But
when they heard it, they went away, one by one, beginning with the eldest, and Jesus was left alone with the
woman standing before him. *Jesus looked up* and said to
her, "Woman, where are they? Has no one condemned
you?" She said, "No one, Lord." And Jesus said, "Neither
do I condemn you; go, and do not sin again."

The first point of vital relevance is philological. This famous
story has formed part of the standard Bible since the fourth century (at the latest), when Jerome decided to absorb it into his
Vulgate Latin text of the Gospel of John, mentioning that he had
found it in "many" Greek and Latin manuscripts. Soon afterward,
Augustine of Hippo wrote his commentary, the *Tractatus in Io-
hannis Evangelium* (413–18? C.E.). However, the *pericope adulterae*
does not appear in the earliest papyrus manuscripts of John. Nor
is it to be found in the crucial third-century manuscripts known
as the Codex Sinaiticus (because it was written in St. Catherine's
Monastery at Mount Sinai), nor the Codex Vaticanus, nor many
other texts and fragments. In fact, the story *does* appear in a few
early manuscripts of Luke, and in some intriguing, rare early
Coptic, Syriac, and Ethiopian translations—which, because they
are so difficult to date, does not help much, except to suggest a
long tradition of oriental adherence and continuity. It may be
that the story originated in Syria some time in the second century C.E., and spread from there.

Elsewhere, in his *De conjugiis adulterinis* (419 C.E.) (2:5),
Augustine tackled head-on the matter of the story's authenticity,
suggesting that one reason for its absence from earlier texts of
John was that it had been suppressed, struck out of their copies
of the Gospel by weak believers, or even enemies of the Church,
who regarded Jesus' treatment of the adulterous woman as mor-
ally lax. These remarks are extraordinarily useful, because they

show that the question of the authenticity of the *pericope adulterae* certainly existed before the earliest reliably datable surviving Greek manuscript "witness" was copied. This appears to be the early-fifth-century Codex Bezae in Cambridge. In fact, John Calvin struck the *pericope adulterae* from *his* edition of the Bible for ostensibly similar reasons, duly fortified by the assumption that it may have been spurious.

The existence of finger imagery of tremendous power in both the Gospels of Luke (the rich man and Lazarus) and of John (doubting Thomas) further complicates the question as to where the *pericope adulterae* might actually "belong," and how much of it was the result of later embellishment. According to the great biblical scholar Raymond E. Brown, the Greek vocabulary seems to be more consistent with Luke than with the author of John. However, the issue remains controversial—because (apart from John) the rudimentary Greek vocabulary of the New Testament does not give textual scholars much to work with.

However, there is a small group of Alexandrian Greek manuscripts, presumably reflecting a relatively early Egyptian textual tradition, that omit the story from John but indicate by means of a pair of dots in the margin, as was the custom, or in one instance by leaving a generous space in the relevant column, either that something was missing in the spot where Jerome thought the story definitely belonged, or else that there was doubt as to whether it or anything else ought to go there at all. This evidence is supremely ambiguous, and the matter is further complicated by the fact that one of the earliest references to the story comes from another Hellenized Egyptian, Didymus the Blind (c. 310/13–c. 395/98 C.E.), who mentioned that he knew the story of the adulteress from "certain gospels," plural. Even so, there is still a minority of scholars who argue "on internal, structural, and external text-critical grounds" that notwithstanding ancient controversy the *pericope adulterae* definitely belongs in John.

The question is important because, as my friend and colleague Andrew McGowan points out, this obviously makes a big difference to the measure of symbolic intensity one should ascribe to the passage. It is axiomatic that the language and imagery of the three Synoptic Gospels tend to be far more straightforward than John: In Mark, Matthew, and Luke a finger might easily just be a finger, and a gloss on the relevant phrase (8:6) in the King James Bible (1611) seems to follow that more prosaic prompt. It reads, plainly, "as if he heard them not." In other words, Jesus ignores the hotheads, keeps his cool, and simply draws lines, or "doodles in the dust."

Yet this certainly did not satisfy the energetic, hugely learned Greek- and Latin-speaking patristic commentators of the early centuries of Christianity. Augustine (33:5) asked: "What else does he signify to you when He writes with His finger on the ground? For the law was written with the finger of God; but written on stone because of the hard-hearted. The Lord now wrote on the ground, because He was seeking fruit." This slightly odd mention of fruit is partly explained by Augustine's careful interpretation of the name of the Mount of Olives (which comes a little earlier, at John 8:1) as meaning "fruitful," "unctuous," and so on, making of it a typically neat Augustinian figure of grace or salvation. "So, fruit is contrasted with stone, as grace with law. Jesus' finger is the finger of God writing the law, as in Exodus."

One of the two central purposes of the episode is to demonstrate Jesus' successful escape from a trap that had been carefully laid for him by the scribes and Pharisees. Jewish religious law, deriving from Moses (and ultimately from those tablets inscribed by the finger of God), was clear on the matter of the woman's adultery, and the challenge to Jesus was either to observe it or publicly to reveal himself to be in dangerous breach. The issue was also of secondary interest to the local Roman authorities, who obviously exercised civil jurisdiction in Palestine, though

as subsequent events were to demonstrate (loudly) this was easily adaptable for expedient political ends. Brilliantly, Jesus turns
the moral and legal problems back upon the consciences of the
woman's accusers, and in this context, as is now usually argued,
the story reflects an increasingly "anti-Jewish" early Christian
standpoint that probably postdates the destruction of the Temple
by the Romans in 70 C.E.

But what did Jesus write with his finger on the ground?
The question recurs, because the text has Jesus stooping to write
twice, once while the trap is being laid, whereupon he stands up
to deliver the key statement "Let him who is without sin . . . ,"
and a second time immediately afterward, as the scribes and
Pharisees drift away, beginning with the oldest (and presumably
wisest, with the largest accumulation of experience). The text
makes a further, vivid allusion to this continuing activity when
it is implied that Jesus is still writing or, at any rate, definitely
still stooping after the crowd has dispersed, the woman is finally
left alone with him, and *he looks up*.

An obvious answer—obvious at least to the glossist in the
ninth-century Vulgate Codex Aureus Monacensis (Munich),
which has a gold cover on which the scene is actually represented—is that as well as speaking the words "Let him who is
without sin . . . ," Jesus actually wrote them out in full. That esoteric iconographical tradition endured right down to Tintoretto
(Rome, Galleria Nazionale dell'Arte Antica), Nicolas Poussin
(Paris, Louvre), Pieter Brueghel the Elder, and other artists who
clearly represented the text at Jesus' feet, rendered in Hebrew—
a solecism. Naturally, there is no internal textual evidence for
this, except for the fact that the action of writing with his finger (maybe the index finger of his right hand; was Jesus right-
handed?) so deliberately brackets the statement in the sequence
of most reliable versions and variants of the text. And textual
sequence is vital because, apart from episodic narrative structure

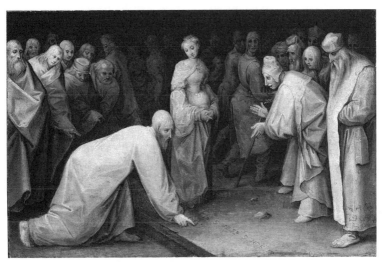

The Brueghels were not especially unusual in imagining Christ writing with his finger on the ground the famous phrase "Let him who is without sin . . . ," but in this case they thought it wise to render Jesus' famous defense of the woman taken in adultery not in words of any ancient language, but rather in contemporary Dutch.

and a thoroughly rudimentary Greek vocabulary, it is largely all we have. But while it is suggestive, it is not enough.

Numerous other patristic commentators of the fourth century, including Hilary (d. 367 c.e.), Ambrosiaster (active 366–84), Ambrose (d. 397), and various other sources, remarked on the story, and a good number joined Augustine in speculating on Jesus' act of writing with his finger on the ground. One gamely suggested that this action alluded to the issue of judgment in general, and to Daniel 5:24 in particular (the original "writing on the wall" in the palace of King Belshazzar). Ambrose is especially sinister, because he imagined Jesus writing out the name of each of the accusers, "that these men have been disowned," apparently a reference to Jeremiah 22:29.

Augustine actually ventured the same opinion (in a second reading, entirely different from the one about law-stone and grace-fruit), but pointed to an earlier passage in Jeremiah for evidence, namely, "O Lord, the hope of Israel, all who forsake you shall be ashamed. Those who depart from me shall be written in the earth, because they have forsaken the Lord, the fountain of the living waters" (17:13). Jerome had referred to the same passage of Jeremiah but felt it could support the even more implausible notion that Jesus wrote out a long and true list of the sins of each of the woman's accusers, which, given the logical constraints of narrative time within the text, would imply that either it was a very short list or that Jesus wrote fast. The suggestion is pure fantasy.

The senses here are robustly anti-Semitic, and further buoyed by hostile glosses elsewhere (as in Eusebius, citing Papias) that suggested the woman was *falsely* accused. In any case, they would appear to be at odds with Jesus' purpose. The reason the episode came under the notice of so many early Christian thinkers at all, apart from rapidly developing anti-Semitism and the question mark that certainly hung over its authenticity, was that through the fourth century the whole question of the duty to forgive versus upholding the law was beginning to cause a headache in the Church and in late antique Roman society, so any model stemming from Jesus himself was plainly relevant. We cannot know what the author of this probably second-century story thought Jesus wrote with his finger on the ground. It is not even certain that this element of the story was not a later embellishment: Didymus' précis (which occurs as an aside in his commentary on the Book of Ecclesiastes) does not even mention the writing, or Jesus' finger. According to the Vulgate text, the scribes and Pharisees heard what Jesus said, but there is absolutely no suggestion that they also read what he wrote. (The Greek verb is unequivocal: *katagraphō*, "to write.") They themselves are obviously silent. The woman probably couldn't read or write. She is silent too. Could this episode have been gratefully committed to memory, and afterward reported by her to the disciples, who were not present, and found its way into the oral tradition by that route? It is conceivable, but we will certainly never know.

The question whether indeed Jesus himself was literate is surprisingly slippery. While John (7:15) tells us that he did not attend what has been called a "high rabbinic school," he was certainly learned. The Jesus of the Gospels knew the Torah inside out, and in childhood showed himself to be that regularly recurring cultural phenomenon, the Jewish wonder child, as is emphasized in Luke (2:41–52). He could apparently recite, that is, *read aloud* from scripture in the Temple (Luke 4:17)—but in ancient Palestine that was not necessarily the same thing as being able to write: Scribes owed their high status to functional literacy, and the Roman provincial tax censuses were good for business; by implication many ordinary Jews either didn't write much, or couldn't at all. Biblical Hebrew was then, as now, an ancient language, not in daily use except liturgically.

According to rabbinical sources of the late second or early third century, at the end of the first century there should have been schools in most Jewish communities, but most probably this does not reflect the basic realities of what was evidently an extremely diverse, multicultural early-first-century Palestine. Apart from using basic Aramaic script to write down your name, for example, or labeling clay jars, and doing other items of simple day-to-day business, even highly numerate tax collectors such as Saul/Paul could apparently survive with relatively basic literacy. In his case, the longest and most complicated Epistles were dictated to a professional scribe (as in Romans 16:22, where he is actually named: Tertius), but Paul claims elsewhere, with uncharacteristic good humor, that while he used very big letters indeed (Galatians 6:11), he wrote at least parts of other Epistles himself. Yet even those statements are misleading because in at least one case (2 Thessalonians 3:17) Paul himself certainly did not compose them. And apart from the standard formulation "it is written," that is, in scripture, there are few other references in the Gospels themselves to the physical act of writing. In Luke (1:63), old Zechariah, the father of John the Baptist, astonishes everybody by writing down on a tablet the name of his baby son. Most other Gospel references are to Moses' "writing" of the law (Mark 10:5 and 12:19; Luke 20:28), and, in John (1:45, 5:47), specifically to Moses' "written" acknowledgment of the coming of the Messiah.

Meanwhile, Geza Vermes has demonstrated how the early-first-century C.E. religious and social elite of Jerusalem and Judea regarded northern Galilean peasants as slow country bumpkins who spoke Aramaic with a strong accent. When, on the eve of the Passion, Peter denied Jesus three times, in fulfillment of the scriptures, it was the Apostle's cloddish Galilean accent that gave him away (Mark 14:70, Luke 22:59, and, even more explicitly, Matthew 26:73). Moreover, Jews from Galilee were thought to have, at best, an imperfect grasp of the Mishnah, the law, scripture, everything. Several passages of the Gospels make explicit reference to this sharp prejudice (Acts 2:13, where in the Pentecost narrative it is presumed that the Galilean disciples were drunk). Even so, it seems unlikely that Jesus had anything more than a few words of Greek, if any at all, and almost certainly no Latin. The idea of a prophet or even the Messiah emerging from the northern provinces was in the aristocratic priestly circle of early-first-century Jerusalem considered at best unlikely, and in spite of the clearly enunciated prophecies of Isaiah (8:23, 9:1), the idea that God should choose to manifest himself in that quarter appears to have been unthinkable.

If the finger of God is a potent recurring image in the Old and New Testaments, its persistence as a powerful echo in the proliferation and veneration of finger relics, and the superstitions attaching to them, has proven remarkably durable throughout the Christian world in the last two thousand years. The index finger of St. John the Baptist was believed to have been miraculously "translated" to the parish church of St. Jean-du-Doigt near Finistère in Brittany during the Hundred Years' War, and its thaumaturgical and miraculous properties were widely celebrated. Not surprisingly, the finger of "Doubting Thomas" is preserved in the church of Santa Croce in Gerusalemme in Rome.

One even encounters related superstitions in the rich harvest of weird provincial lore patiently accumulated by those invaluable and dogged Victorian antiquarians. In 1864, for example, the correspondent of *Trewman's Exeter Flying Post* reported at length a strange story about the vault of a prominent local family, that of M—— (in ——shire), on which there was the figure of a kneeling angel carved in white marble, "with one hand and finger pointing upward." According to the old gray sexton, Mr. Judkin,

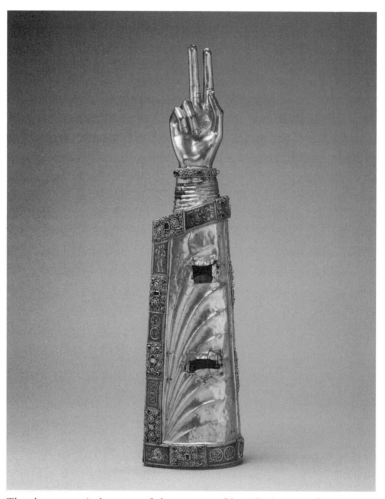

The thaumaturgical power of the gesture of benediction was for centuries enhanced by the orchestration in reliquary containers of the arm and finger bones of dead saints.

Before any of the family of the M—— die the angel is
seen to move for a moment downward the uplifted finger. If you smile at the superstition he [the sexton] will
give you dates for these coincidences, and will declare
that he himself, on more occasions than one, beheld
the angel's finger move, when a death in the old gabled
manor house invariably followed. "The old squire," he
said, "the last before the present one, was in the family
pew at morning service, and in sound health, when with
his own eyes he saw the angel's finger move. He told me
himself; for I overtook him after locking the church, on
his way to the house, and he said, 'Judkin, there is one
of us that has got the summons. I saw the angel's finger
move, as the parson was preaching.'" After this the sexton looks you in the face and adds, "the summons was
for the squire hisself; he died of 'plexy on the following
Saturday evening, an hour before bed-time."

Though infrequently isolated in the canonical Gospels, the
finger of God and subsidiary fingers vividly operating in the
supernatural realm have proven durable symbols of divine imminence, but it is in the Eastern religions with which we began
that one finds its almost infinite capacity for eloquence amply
exploited. Mudras, from the Sanskrit word that means literally
"seal" or "signet"—as impressed in wax for securing old letters
to guarantee their integrity and privacy, or affixed to official documents as proof of authenticity—are mostly gestures of the hand
and fingers that enjoy a long and uninterrupted history in Hinduism and Buddhism in their many branches, and a concomi-
tant importance in the iconographical traditions associated with
particular religious practices, spiritual attitudes, and indeed states
of being. Mudras are an essential ingredient of traditional Hindu
dance. They are an essential component of the practice and disci-

pline of meditation. They are variously associated with carefully
differentiated deities, bodhisattvas, or conditions of enlightenment or "buddhahood." And their complex evolving meanings,
often highly specific, are to be statically observed above all in
the attitude of hands and finger gestures in the great traditions
of South and East Asian figural sculpture. As the Englishman
Monier Monier-Williams put it in his sketchy, Raj-minded *Hinduism* of 1877, presumably for the benefit of perplexed mem-
sahibs who might otherwise have wondered, "The term *Mudrā*
is also used in Tāntrism to denote mystical intertwinings of the
fingers so as to form symbolical figures."

According to Emeritus Professor Fredrick W. Bunce of Indiana State University, whose exhaustive and authoritative catalog was recently published in New Delhi, the many hundreds of
documented mudras may be divided into four principal subcategories:

> (1) those which are generally held or depicted in the rep-
> resentation of deities, demigods, godlings, demons, and
> heroes, both Buddhist and Hindu; (2) those which are
> associated with particular *tantric* worship, particularly of
> Japanese, Chinese, and Tibetan *Vajrayana* or *Matrayana* rites
> [the "thunderbolt" tantric rites of Mahayana Buddhism
> and the "mantra"-oriented rites respectively]; (3) those
> which are associated with *yogic* meditational practices . . .

and, finally, (4) those employed in theater and dance, which often replicate or exploit the fame of mudras belonging to the
other three. The first category is relatively restricted to dozens
of mudras only, and are, on the whole, much confined to "static"
or single-handed (*asamyutta*) positions, although two-handed
(*samyutta*) mudras, some of them important, are occasionally also
connected with supernatural beings. Likewise, single-handed

mudras are employed in the remaining three categories, which are generally adopted or enacted by living people, though it is the double-handed mudras that here predominate, and occasionally require carefully choreographed movements also. Within the enormous literature on this subject there are four interlocking problems of interpretation. The Sanskrit, Tibetan, Mandarin, Cantonese, Mongolian, Korean, and Japanese languages (at various stages in their history and development) do not always clearly describe particular, often intricate gestures. This is hardly surprising given their range. On at least one occasion, 1,811 separate illustrations have been needed to cover the subject in Japan alone. The fact that most mudras are formed by interposing, positioning, combining, or swiveling at the wrist, the nearly universal quota of ten fingers can cause great confusion.

Second, there is a considerable amount of repetition and duplication in form but distinctive variations in usage throughout the Hindu and Buddhist worlds. One mudra can mean very different things on opposite sides of the Himalayas, while it follows that identically the same concept can obviously be indicated by mudras that from place to place are completely unalike.

Third, visual evidence can at times be poorly drafted or drawn and at times enshrines a genuine misunderstanding of the early written sources and traditions: Do we try to follow the descriptions, or trust the interpretative drawings that illustrate them in old books and manuscripts? How does the three-dimensional evidence of surviving sculpture cleave to either one? At least one desperate diagrammist attempted to solve this problem by contriving a left hand happily equipped with a thumb and five other fingers, so hopelessly did the written description of this particular mudra tie him up in knots.

Finally, local politics have from time to time created difficulties as, for example, when King Rama III established forty mudras that were deemed by him and his religious advisers acceptable for Thai representations of the postures of the Lord Buddha, bringing the total number of these to at least fifty-eight. These include apostrophized positions and attitudes that stood in for "cutting his topknot," "undergoing austerities," "accepting an offering of honey-sweetened rice," "looking at the Bodhi tree in gratefulness," "partaking of a myrobalan nut," "reflecting," "pacifying the ocean," "persuading the relatives not to quarrel," "giving pardon or dispelling fear" (as distinct from "blessing"), "contemplating the truth of aging," performing various cosmic marvels and miracles, and "reclining and entering *parinirvana*." Not many of these closely adhere to traditional Hindu or Buddhist mudras of earlier centuries, and the Thai names applied to ones that do are often unrelated to any surviving Indic terminology. Mudras are nothing if not complicated, and this is, of course, a substantial part of their charm.

Indeed, mudras can be wholly esoteric, denoting an almost infinite number of degrees of specific meaning that may more or less readily conform to the visual effect. For example, the *dharmachakra* mudra is relatively common in the Buddhist tradition. "It denotes preaching by setting the wheel of the law into motion." The tips of the thumb and index finger touch; the middle, ring, and little fingers are extended; and this pose is held in both hands, the palms facing each other at close quarters but not touching. The positions of the hands are slightly unequal in height, but held at roughly chest level. "This mudrā is generally associated with the Lord Buddha, but also *Vairochana* and *Maitreya*."

Vairochana (more often Vairocana or Mahāvairocana) is a "Buddha concept" held to embody the universal qualities of the original Gautama Buddha, and in a different sense the aspirational Buddha concept of "emptiness," for which living devotees strive. Maitreya, by contrast, is an eschatological Buddha concept, in other words, the Buddha who will come at the end of time and impart the otherwise unattainable teachings of perfection. That both should be regularly, even commonly represented adopting the *dharmachakra* mudra, and emulated by living persons who understand the full implication of that gesture, packs a powerful theological punch.

In an entirely different context the *nalini-padmakosha* mudra is the special province of the actor or dancer, and simply indicates buds or clusters of flowers. The palms face outward; the fingers and thumbs are gently adducted and flexed, and therefore curve gracefully toward the palms without touching them. Thus positioned, the hands are crossed at the wrists. The *kamjayi* mudra, meanwhile, belongs to the yogic tradition, and involves the right hand only. The palm faces out; the index finger curls back and its tip rests below the nail of the thumb. Likewise, the middle finger curls back and its tip rests on the second knuckle of the index finger; the ring finger follows suit, the tip resting on the second knuckle of the middle finger, while—and no doubt you can see this coming—the little finger orients itself identically in respect to the second knuckle of the ring finger. "So formed, the mudrā is held chest-high." Easier said than done. If you can ever manipulate your hand into this uncomfortable, actually impossible mudra—it is obviously best to start practicing when you are very young—you might be surprised to discover that in the Yoga Tatva Mudra Vigyan form of yoga this mudra is used to repress sexual urges. I have no doubt whatsoever that it is very effective.

Perhaps one of the most famous and immediately recognizable mudras for Western observers because of its magnificent use in related Burmese and Thai statues of the Lord Buddha is the *bhumisparsha* mudra, which is actually very widespread throughout Asia. The mudra involves both hands, and is held by the Buddha while seated and meditating. The right forearm rests on the right thigh. The hand is relaxed and bends at the wrist, and the fingers point downward (frequently touching the ground), presenting to the observer the dorsal side of the hand. The left hand is relaxed and rests in the lap, supine, palm facing upward (in fact another, separate mudra, the *dhyana*). By this combined gesture the Lord Buddha calls the earth to witness the defeat of evil forces represented by Mara, the Hindu god of pestilence and mortal disease, an accomplishment he attained during the famous forty-day meditation under the Bodhi tree. In its calm eloquence, grace, and simplicity, the performance of "calling the earth to witness" is to my mind one of the most incomparably beautiful of all Buddhist attitudes, no less moving for the fact that in this iteration the motions of the fingers of each divine hand are subdued without permitting them to sprawl or merely dangle. If there is a good lesson to be learned from Buddhist spirituality, it is that here, as elsewhere, calm and concentration, relaxation and self-control, great eloquence and total silence, go hand in hand.

FOUR

The Finger and Communication

...an *Ancient Clearke*, skilfull in Presidents, Wary in Proceeding, and Vnderstanding in the *Businesse* of the *Court*, is an excellent Finger of a *Court*; And doth many times point the way to the *Iudge* himselfe.

—Sir Francis Bacon, *Essay 56: Of Iudicature* (1625)

My earliest memory, as vivid to me now as if it were yesterday, is the sight of a shaft of afternoon sunlight falling against the back of a pair of closed curtains in the old nursery. Those curtains were decorated with leaping black horses, and maybe a few small Chinese characters also, widely spaced against a buff-colored background, and I once had the startling experience of seeing an eerily similar design at the Metropolitan Museum of Art in New York, to which clearly most if not all aesthetic roads eventually lead. I am pointing at the horses and the sunlight through the wooden rails surrounding my cot. My mother is there too. She must have come in to open the curtains, and get me up from my nap, but what stands out is that bright shaft of strong southern light slanting over the back of the curtains, and those leaping black horses.

For an infant, pointing is the key to the acquisition of language, the "royal road" to speech, as the late George Butterworth so memorably put it. Obviously, from about the age of a few months babies can point with the index finger at anything, anytime they choose, but what makes this gesture so useful for learning language is when it conforms to three basic circumstances. First, it is a way of attracting the attention of someone else to the object of shared interest or curiosity: Look at that. What is it? Building on this, the baby can by this means isolate that thing from all the other surrounding curiosities, and background noise, and to focus for a moment on what makes that thing different from all the others. Look at that. What is it *specifically*? Finally, the gesture of pointing is almost invariably outward-moving, a projection away from the baby's own body, often scatter-gun certainly, but (rather like the smile at a much earlier stage of development) a crucial acknowledgment of the baby's rapidly accumulating and deepening awareness of the sharp division between the emerging self and the world. Look at that. Whatever it is, I want it for myself. All parents know what squalls may ensue when the baby discovers that that hotly desired thing is not yet available.

Now, what is so fascinating about babies' discovery of pointing with the index finger is that it seems to be partly learned but also partly innate. In other words, at about the age of six months babies become fully aware of pointing in adults, and fully comprehend the attention-getting purpose of that gesture, and indeed duly focus on the shared object of contemplation, a good two months or so (on average) before they start pointing with vigor themselves. By the time this happens babies have already begun to recognize and respond to the names of objects and people, so in a sense the processes of pointing-wanting, pointing-naming, and pointing-learning are driven by the urgent necessity to extend and accumulate, rather than to build absolutely from scratch. And these are powerfully tied to vision. Pointing gestures do not come so readily or so early to the congenitally blind. Above all, pointing with the index finger appears to be

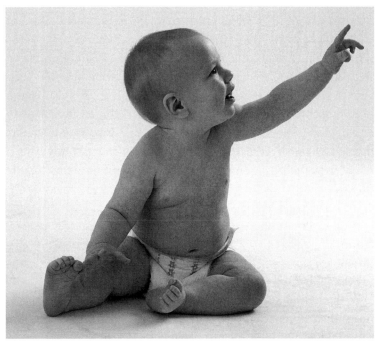

Far more than a universal method of indication, for babies, pointing with the index finger is the key to the rapid development of language itself.

"biologically based, and species specific"; closely related to the development of left- or right-handedness; and likewise a vital stage toward the discovery of precision grip. Look at that. Not only do I want it for myself; I shall go ahead and feel, hold, and, if possible, *take* it. Many strings of pearls have come adrift as a result of this remarkable and rapid sequence of developmental steps, and upon the vestigial remnants of this vital infantile hunger for knowledge, grasping, and possession the whole apparatus of modern marketing depends for its remarkable ability to revive and deploy it in adults for commercial gain. With luck we spend the rest of our lives learning what not to want, and how to get rid of material possessions, but clearly many of us fail to acquire that skill.

The cultural history of gesture is, of course, a vast field, and getting vaster. In one sense the burgeoning interest in nonverbal communication that characterizes many historical and scientific disciplines just now runs parallel with the gradual decline of many highly sophisticated gesturing practices that once flourished all over the world. Some cultures still use many types of gesture far more than others, and nobody who has ever spent any amount of time living in Italy has not noticed the persistence of numerous, highly specific attitudes of the hands that remain firmly embedded in Italian language and culture—from the upraised hand with conjoined fingertips (all five) that accompanies *"ma dai"* or *"che vuoi?"* (the equivalent of "come on" or "what do you want?" or "you *must* be joking"), through the *corni* by which the superstitious seek to ward off the evil eye (index and little fingers extended; middle and ring fingers folded onto the palm; the equivalent of our "fingers crossed"), to the index finger of one hand planted firmly downward and perpendicularly onto the palm of the other, which says *"insisto!"* Rather more sinister is the *minaccia*, the explicit threat—a slashing motion with the flat of the hand across the throat whose meaning is unmistakable.

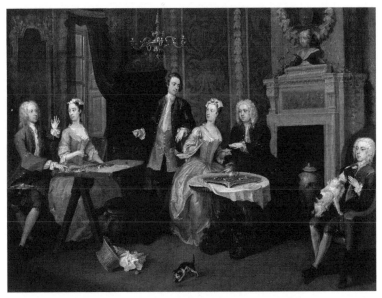

In Hogarth's mysterious family drama, glances and declamation revolve around the demonstrative index finger of the standing young gentleman, whose handkerchief the seated hostess is surreptitiously removing from his pocket with the thumb and index finger of her right hand.

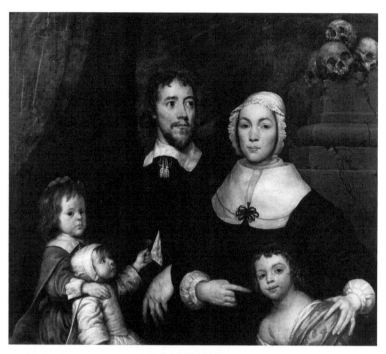

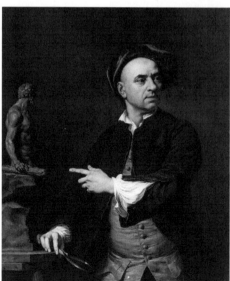

The universality of pointing with the index finger: In Dobson's portrait, Mrs. Streatfield memorializes her dead son, while John Michael Rysbrack proudly acknowledges the clay model for his famous statue of Hercules.

The task, then, of accumulating gestures with particular significance is as huge as that of compiling dictionaries of spoken and written languages, but hampered at times by a fundamental lack of precision in the sources—the same problem attending mudras. However, this has not deflected many specialist scholars who, driven by curiosity and exhibiting remarkable *Sitzfleisch*, have patiently gone ahead and compiled enormous compendia in which to preserve the vanishing languages of gesture that once thrived in many societies and periods, for example among silent orders of Trappist and Cistercian monks. Indeed, formal sign languages also once flourished among tribal peoples of different language groups who nevertheless required a convenient method of communicating with one another over relatively short geographical distances. This was especially the case among Australian Aborigines, the peoples of the highlands and coastal plains of Papua New Guinea, and many First Nations Americans, for all of whom systematic languages of gesture also came to fulfill a ritual storytelling and religious function, extending far beyond the practicalities that gave rise to those languages in the first place—comparing notes about hunting and scouting, for example; checking and agreeing upon the different phases of the moon; waging war, or suing for peace. There have always been sign languages for the benefit of the deaf and mute, but sometimes there have been ritual bans on speech—temporary or even occasionally permanent—that made species of gesture not only necessary but indispensable. Not all of them were monastic in nature; married Armenian women in the Caucasus were prevented by convention from speaking to their husbands' male relatives, and solved the problem by adopting a convenient language of gesture. Finally, there is the astonishing proliferation of gesture languages that have developed for dramatic effect in many traditions of dance and theater, a powerful embellishment of the spoken word, and at times also a source of fine syntactical tuning within the broad aesthetic framework of choreography.

Prayer and benediction; magic and incantation; practicalities
such as distance (sailors, surveyors, sports referees); noise (workers
in steel mills, firemen, pilots); confidentiality (spies and criminals,
pitchers and catchers, auctioneers); the overriding requirement
of silence (experienced most obviously by the conductors of
orchestras; although, delightfully, one may still hear the voice of
Sir Thomas Beecham in a few rare recordings saying "Louder!");
or even, as we shall see later, the conventions of driving on a
road or highway—the one thing that all of these situations share
is that for whatever reason gesture takes the place of speech,
and functions separately as a form of language, sometimes crude
or basic, but often highly sophisticated. There are scholars of
linguistics who have also sought to isolate certain universals: in
other words, a repertoire of biologically encoded expressions of
fear and anxiety that cause us to take up the prompt, as it were,
of the infant's pointing gesture with the index finger, and irre-
sistibly apply it to speech—far beyond the most basic indicators
of, for example, *you, me, up, down, here, there, thirsty,* and *sex,* that
have, after all, since the dawn of time enabled us humans rapidly
to confront the problem of, first, encountering a language other
than our own, then by trial and error deciphering and learning
it. To all these ends our fingers are an obviously indispensable
vocabulary, semaphore, toolbox, wand, typewriter, instruction
manual, alarm bell, and megaphone rolled into one.

Three principal examples will serve to illustrate the awesome-
ness of these phenomena. I have a strong personal attachment to
St. Odo, the second abbot of the great Benedictine monastery
of Cluny, because lately I found that prayers fervently addressed
to him in his capacity as patron saint of lost property are powerfully effective. However, it is as a capable administrator of his
monastery that St. Odo concerns us here, for the abbot imposed
"such a strict rule of silence upon his brethren" that if one were
to communicate at all it became necessary to employ a system

of signs. That system took root and found ample nourishment in tenth-century Cluny, and, leaving aside the question of whether such a formal language of gesture actually served to bypass the very rule of silence that was intended to define the spiritual atmosphere of the community but at the same time made it exceedingly difficult to function at all—because it soon emerged that some monks using the in-house sign language were as chatty, garrulous, and prone to gossip as they would have been if they were allowed to speak—eventually for the benefit of postulants and novices it became essential to codify and standardize the system.

Udalricus of Cluny compiled lists of gestures for this purpose, and William of Hirschau subsequently helped himself to the original list and freshened it up. From both we now know what contingencies the sign language of Cluny was designed to cover, but unfortunately we do not know exactly what all the corresponding signs and gestures were like. Certainly individual hand signals were adopted for "different sorts of bread, vegetables, fish, fruit, other comestibles, spices, liquids, vases, vestments, liturgical objects, ordinary books, different sorts of people (from peasant to bishop), buildings, tools and implements, 'and other things as well.'"

From the rudimentary descriptions given in Latin for many of these gestures it seems that the practices of Cluny coincided in many respects with similar conventions used by the Cistercians. After all, there was no reason for one order of monks to reinvent the wheel when another had already taken the trouble of doing so. Indeed, the advantage of a shared, intermonastic language of gesture was that it facilitated contact between monk-scholars seeking to copy manuscripts in one another's libraries—though it is impossible to imagine that from time to time monks did not, out of sheer frustration, break into full-throated Latin, to navigate some semantic point so hopelessly beyond the capacity of the gesture system to convey.

There are some baffling anomalies, such as the fact that in Cluny the specific gesture for "trout," which seems to have involved some sort of rippling fishy motion of the hand, also meant "woman," a bizarre convergence that is only partly explained by the fact that it derived from the fall of a distinctive type of veil or headdress commonly worn by Frenchwomen in the tenth and eleventh centuries. Within the cloistered environment I suppose the context usually made it clear whether you meant "trout" or "woman." Technically, Benedictine monks were not allowed to catch, clean, gut, fillet, and then fry a woman; nevertheless, at least some potential for considerable confusion, even embarrassment, must have existed.

Another drawback of the system was that occasionally monks invented fake signs, out of mischief, to sabotage the conversation, to run rings around the novices, or deliberately to create the false impression that they possessed immense and arcane learning. Meanwhile at Canterbury in the twelfth century, Giraldus Cambrensis was astonished to observe a riotous commotion at mealtime in the refectory, where the monks (who as fellow Benedictines were by then also using the sign language of Cluny) were both gesticulating wildly and whispering audibly and angrily, fully confident that both sets of actions satisfactorily flew under the radar of the ban on plain speech. And in those silent communities that still existed in the twentieth century, the problem of adapting a centuries-old medieval system to the requirements of modern life and commerce evidently led to the formulation of ingenious compound gestures such as "bull" and "push" for earthmoving equipment, "cold" and "house" for refrigerator, and the complicated sequence of "thank," "God," "day," and "bird" for turkey.

The remarkable thing about the monastic sign languages was that they were adopted more or less voluntarily. No such latitude has ever existed for the deaf. There is ample evidence that deaf people have always developed and used for themselves and those nearest to them a set of effective signing conventions, and the question in the minds of eighteenth- and nineteenth-century pioneers of a more formal system of sign language was whether these gestures constituted some sort of *"langage des signes naturelles"* (language of natural signs), reflecting, in other words, an innate capacity to reach within and produce a range of shared "pantomimic" gestures upon which a more formal language might be built. The gestures routinely employed by "primitive" peoples were thoroughly investigated with this question at least partly in mind, and mixed conclusions reached. However, in 1750, Charles Michel, abbé de l'Épée, was convinced that, even if such a universal repertoire of signs and hand signals could be shown to exist, it was clearly inadequate to describe or encapsulate many abstract concepts. Over the ensuing decades he set about creating a methodical language of signs, which culminated in the publication in Paris in 1776 of his *L'Institution des sourds et muets par la voie des signes méthodiques*, something of a breakthrough, and the start of a tremendous movement toward equipping the deaf and mute with the ability to communicate with one another and with the rest of us on as equal and as standardized a footing as possible—or at least far less unequal than before it and related sign languages were taken up all over the world.

The project of the ambitious abbé de l'Épée in fact took two forms. Supported by a substantial inheritance, he aimed to create a special school in Paris for the deaf-mute, and to develop a universal sign language, that is, not a version of French but a new language of gesture that would serve to bridge the communication gap principally among the deaf themselves, and between his pupils and himself. And he developed this through years of more or less successful experimentation. Maddeningly, the earliest publication of his method—which was methodical only in the sense that it was subject to rules laid down by him—

contains no illustrations, and does not really give us an accurate idea of what the new sign language was like. However, the abbé claimed he was careful to incorporate as many and as practical a range of gestures as were proffered by the pupils themselves, a nod toward the old idea of the innateness of deaf-mute gesturing. Upon this bedrock he aimed to solidify abstract meanings, "determine proper usage," standardize and impose upon the growing repertoire a systematic grammar, devise suitable methods of indicating tense, gender, and even a six-case sequence of declensions. To this he gradually added elements of what we would now call speech therapy: lipreading and other aids that at first he rejected as being too time-consuming and fraught with difficulty and frustration, but later came to realize were the only ways for his pupils successfully to communicate with the outside world, and with people who did not and would obviously never know their unique, in-house language of signs. An initial commitment to and faith in the potential for a new and universal sign language for use by deaf people among themselves was eventually therefore replaced by the insight that in order to build any kind of avenue of communication, deaf people needed to be able to understand and speak French (as best they could). The way forward was therefore for the new language of gesture and spoken language to merge, and this is precisely what has happened, step by step, since the abbé de l'Épée first opened his school in the rue des Moulins, and in most other places where conventions of sign language for the deaf now prosper.

Many formal sign languages, including those specifically developed for the deaf, combine up to five distinct types of gesture, many but by no means all chiefly confined to the hands and fingers. Pantomimic signs aim to reproduce the action for which they stand, or the object they represent—such as the index and middle fingers extended and set in motion to mimic the action of walking, or else the tips of the thumb and index and middle fingers joined and raised to the mouth to indicate eating. Pure signs, so-called, are by contrast signs that bear no direct resemblance to the action or thing that they represent, but nevertheless carry a specific meaning. The color terminology of the Cistercians was largely confined to pure signs of this type: yellow, for instance, was indicated with the tips of the index and middle fingers of the right hand by tracing a line from between your eyebrows down the bridge of your nose to the tip. Although the action has no visible connection with the concept of yellow, nevertheless that is what it meant to the Cistercians. "Qualitative signs" were especially useful for indicating nationalities and places, and did so by assigning characteristics that served to identify each by association. Rome, for example, was indicated by combining gestures for "Pope" and "courtyard"; Africa, "black" and "courtyard"; and latterly, Russia, "red" and "courtyard"; and so on. Further subgroups combined gestures of these different types to form new abstract concepts, either bypassing the corresponding conventions of speech or else actually referencing them directly. And ultimately a systematized set of specific finger gestures for the letters of the alphabet, including useful contractions and abbreviations borrowed from the various older subcategories, came to dominate sign language for the deaf. The most important point to grasp about these interlocking strategies is the degree to which they may either adhere very closely to the conventions of formal language or else diverge radically from it, yet the combined effect is to replace the audibility of the spoken word with the visibility and clarity of gesture.

In current American Sign Language, and other cognate sign languages for the deaf, some gestures refer explicitly to the distinctive shape and disposition of the roman letters for which they stand, for example, *D* (index finger extended, middle, ring and little fingers opposed—which actually approximates a small *d*); I (the little finger raised); *O* (the thumb opposed to the index and middle fingers, the remaining two flexing in unison); *L* (the thumb and index finger fully extended); *V* (for "victory"), and *Z* (for which the index finger traces a zigzag). Others have no such direct correspondence with the equivalent letter: for example, *B* (the index through little fingers extended, thumb folded onto palm); *H* (the index and middle fingers extended; thumb folded over ring and little fingers); or *E* (the second to fifth fingertips all brought to rest on the back of the folded thumb). But somewhat like the system of pictograms upon which the Chinese languages are built, or the use in Japanese of four entirely different sets of characters (kanji, hiragana, katakana, and romaji), American Sign Language also embraces gestures that stand for whole concepts as well, which condenses what would otherwise require much tedious finger spelling into the eloquence of a single flourish, stroke, or pat. In other words, taken together with lipreading, this and similar systems of sign language attack the problem of nonverbal communication on numerous fronts simultaneously.

In these situations the hands and fingers are the indicators of meaning, but when in 1824, at the remarkably early age of fifteen, Louis Braille began to adapt and simplify for the benefit of blind people an overly complicated phonetic system of "night writing," originally developed for confidential communication between soldiers on the battlefield, the finger became a powerful reader instead. The original system was the brainchild of Charles Barbier de la Serre, and required the use of two columns of up to six dots that corresponded with the coordinates of a thirty-six-cell grid on which all the letters of the alphabet and the commonest diphthongs and letter sequences in French were plotted. The problem was that reading it required first grasping the two-digit coordinates, then decoding each in turn, and gradually accumulating the meaning of whole words. Barbier did his best to arrange the grid so that the simplest coordinates corresponded with the commonest letters and vowels, but the higher numerical coordinates such as 6-5 and 5-6 were easily confused, and difficult to remember. Braille's principal idea—the root of its brilliance—was that there were too many dots, and no direct equivalence to individual letters. Instead he devised a combination of up to six raised dots arranged in two columns of three, each combination of one, two, three dots, and so on, corresponding with letters of the alphabet and numerals, and in due course even musical notation. The basic proportion of Braille's grid of only six dots meant that each letter could be distinguished much more easily from the rest, and by the tip of one finger only.

This was not the first form of writing for the blind. Indeed, up to the end of the eighteenth century many blind people were able to teach themselves to read from printed books relying entirely upon the slight indentation of the metal type on sufficiently heavy paper, and to develop any number of other remarkable manual and musical skills, usually working in isolation. Diderot marveled at the various accomplishments of the young Mademoiselle de Salignac, who, though blind,

> wrote with a pin, with which she pricked a sheet of paper, stretched upon a frame: on this were placed two moveable metal rods, having a sufficient space between them, in which to form the letters. The same mode of writing was adopted in answering her letters, which she read by passing her fingers over the inequalities made by the pin, on the reverse of the paper. She could read a book printed on one side only, and Priault printed some in this manner for her use.

Later, systems of embossed roman lettering were adopted for use by blind people, but naturally these were clumsy, difficult to circulate, and nearly impossible to use. As with all truly great inventions, Braille's writing system had the virtue of simplicity, and moreover took advantage of the extreme sensitivity of a single fingertip without taxing the blind reader by too complex or numerous an arrangement of dots.

The sheer power of the simple gesture of pointing with the index finger may be gauged by its long and remarkably per-sistent use as an aide memoire by the enthusiastic readers and annotators of manuscripts, documents, and printed books since the Renaissance (at the latest). This fascinating story has been set out in detail lately by William H. Sherman, and it emerges that the "fist" (a misnomer), or manicule, as he calls it, a tiny draw-ing of a disembodied hand with elongated index finger—often hugely elongated —was routinely drawn in the margin to note words, phrases, or passages of vital importance, or merely to note something of passing interest. Beyond the simple mar-ginal note or sidelining, or the use of more abbreviated marks such as the distant ancestors of the asterisk, exclamation point, and question mark, many Renaissance readers took the time and trouble carefully to inscribe manicules as well. Some are stubby and crude. Others imply by the strength of their line, and the sharpness of their disposition, a corresponding measure of criti-cal acuity in the draftsman. Occasionally, authors themselves used manicules to lay particular, even overriding emphasis upon a point or passage, but obviously not by those whose intellectual vanity prevented them from doing so on the grounds that such strong emphasis might better be laid by means of language alone. In any event, the manicule passed gracefully into print—and indeed has since flourished in dictionaries and encyclopedias, particularly as a cross-referencing device. A stylish version with jagged cuff originally designed in the 1890s by Will Bradley for the Ameri-can Typefounders Company remains in widespread use.

As if to remind us of the long thread of continuity that joins interested readers and laboring writers of every age, the direct descendant of all these manicule devices still hovers eerily over your computer screen, the index finger extended, the thumb patiently standing by, the other three folded over—and three little vertical lines indicate that it is unequivocally the back of the hand that we are looking at and not the palm, a satisfactory nod toward the relevant tendons, or maybe rows of stitches on some notional glove. There are sadly not enough pixels to be absolutely sure of this point, but one of the curious and delightful things about images is that occasionally we see only what we know, instead of what others urge us to see.

FIVE

The Finger and the Economy

She shows that wives are wont to be selected more on the basis of
wealth than of character and that many are guided, not by their eyes, but
by their fingers, in marrying.

—St. Jerome, *Adversus Jovinianum* (392–93 C.E.), 1:46

Just as the gesture of pointing provides each infant with one of
the most important tools for the acquisition of language, the
system of numbering to the power of ten that we share with
many cultures across diverse historical periods probably originated with what our distant ancestors found at their fingertips.
There have been important exceptions, such as counting to the
power of twenty (fingers and toes), or twelve (fingers and two
feet; or else the joints of four fingers minus the thumb), and more
primitive counting systems developed around the concepts of
two (hands), four (hands and feet), five (the fingers of one hand),
and, intriguingly, eight, a rare anomaly once encountered among
a certain group of First Nations Americans, which, according to
John D. Barrow, owes its existence not to the fingers themselves
but the spaces separating them—four on each hand.

Though by definition entirely undocumented, the prehistory
of numbers is nevertheless a rich field for speculation and conjec-
ture. Certainly the strength of the finger hypothesis derives from
its inherent logic. The challenge for the modern historian seems

to be more squarely to prove an alternative origin of counting to the power of ten, and to positively discount the fingers as its source, than actually to defend it. This is, I think, because the close relationship between number and finger is powerfully reinforced by an equally ancient, if not innate tendency to use the digits for all kinds of other mnemonic and poetic purposes that run parallel with counting. It is very common to observe someone accumulating the points of an argument by counting them off on the fingers of one hand by using the index finger of the other; rather less common when those points exceed five—or the arguer lacks concision, is prone to losing his train of thought, or is liable to drift down byways. In any case, our ancestors freely availed themselves of the list-making usefulness of the fingers—to catalog the vices of the devil, as we saw in the beginning; to parse the stages of life; or as a convenient method of remembering which months of the year have thirty-one days, and which do not. This intriguing device was observed in rural Holland in the 1890s by that attentive traveler and accumulator of lore, customs, and bons mots Henry Attwell:

> The knuckles of the hand represent months of thirty-one days, and the spaces between represent months of thirty days. Thus, the first knuckle is January (thirty-one), the first space February (twenty-eight or twenty-nine, the exception), the second knuckle March (thirty-one), the second space April (thirty), &c. The fourth knuckle, July (thirty-one), is followed by the first [i.e., of the same hand], August (thirty-one), and so on, until the third knuckle is reached a second time. This sequence of two knuckles [i.e., fourth followed by first] corresponds with the only sequence of months (July and August) which have each thirty-one days. This *memoria tecnica* certainly gives a more ready result than the rhyme ["Thirty Days Hath September . . ."].

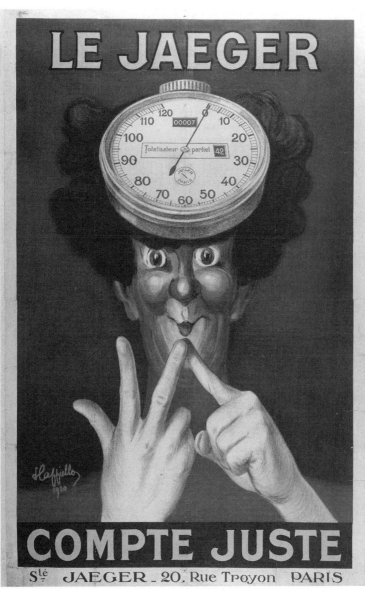

To counting with the fingers we may attribute the obscure origin of counting to the power of ten, though in this case the point was harnessed cheerfully (if rather strangely) to emphasize the accuracy of Jaeger timepieces.

Yet the mnemonic function of the fingers is curiously back-and-forth in character, because there is also a rich folkloric tradition of naming them for their own sake, and by this ingenious method impressing upon children at various stages of development the essentially indexical character of the fingers, and their vast potential for numerical, placeholding, and other uses. These days doting parents and others might play the game of "eeny, meeny, miney, mo" upon their children's digits, but this practice is exceedingly ancient, and yields many memorable variants—indeed, that they were so memorable is certain proof of their efficacy. People who spent their early childhood in late Regency Shropshire and Cheshire, for example, long afterward still remembered learning to name their fingers with the following nursery mantra:

> Thumb, Tommy Tompkins.
> First finger, Billy Wilkins.
> Second finger, Long Larum.
> Third finger, Betsy Bedlam.
> Fourth finger, Little Bob.

A variant of this ran

> Tom Thumbkin,
> Bill Witkin,
> Long Lorum,
> Bessie Borum,
> And the little boy that runs on before 'em.

A slightly more worrying Nottinghamshire version of the same formula was

> Tom Thumper,
> Ben Bumper,

Long 'nation,
Tem'tation,
Little man o' war, war, war!

In Scotland the same practice was quite different again, and distinctly gloomier. In the 1940s, an old Englishwoman recalled that in the light of a flickering candle her Scottish nurse recited the tally of fingers thus:

Thumb, Black Barney;
Finger, Lope Dake;
Finger, Steel Corney;
Finger, Runaway;
And Little Canny Wanny who Pays All,

while a different Scottish source gave

This is the man who broke the barn:
This is the man who stole the cow:
This is the man who stood and saw:
This is the man who ran awa'
And wee peeriwinkie paid for a'.

Several of these schemes appear to account for the activities of four bucolic thieves—sometimes a single one—concluding with the little finger that must stoically bear the cost. A closely related form survived in Lancashire, but omitted the thumb, and casts the little finger as a fugitive:

This broke the barn,
This stole the corn,
This got none:
This went pinky-winky all the way home!

These naming conventions sometimes crossed over into the strange but longstanding practices of divination and fortune-telling. Depending upon whether they appeared on the thumb or on the index, middle, ring, or little finger, "the white specks which occasionally appear on the finger-nails" were in some Edwardian nurseries firmly believed to predict

A gift,
A beau,
A friend,
A foe, or
A voyage to go.

The practice of indicating with the fingers not merely the numerals 1 to 10, but all numbers from one up to ten thousand, was firmly established in ancient Egypt, Sumeria, and Babylon, where the physical world was first divided into 360 geometrical degrees, directly relating to measurements of time into 360 days per year (an ingenious, but sadly inaccurate calculation), and further subdivisions into sixty minutes per hour, and sixty seconds per minute. This framework has regularly been ascribed to a fundamental ancient Babylonian count of the thirty finger joints of both hands (including the first metacarpals, that is, those supporting the thumbs). Whether or not you follow this mighty effort to account for the standardized measurements of time and space in the ancient Near East, it seems clear that the structure of the digits—even the tally of knuckles and intervening gaps between them (seven, not including the thumb, which in this case acted as a kind of accountant or enumerator)—provided a powerfully suggestive prompt that enabled early philosophers to order the world partly according to the structure of the human body, specifically the hand.

Counting with the aid of complex finger gestures became

so sophisticated and widespread in the ancient Roman Republic—where you could cogently count up to one million using the fingers of both hands—that the many references to its component gestures are almost impossible to decipher for the simple reason that later authors such as Seneca, Tertullian, Pliny the Younger, Ambrose, and Augustine assumed that everyone knew what they were talking about. Certainly the English word *digit*, meaning each of the numerals below 10, originated with the Latin word for finger, which also doubled as a Roman unit of measurement; that is, a *digitus* was one sixteenth of a *pes*, or foot. The ancient Greeks worked with an identical concept; the *daktylos* (finger) was one sixteenth of a *pous* (foot), though both Greek measurements were a fraction larger than their Roman equivalents. However, as regards the formal system of counting with the fingers, the sources can be woefully obscure. In an aside in his second-century *Apologia*, for example, the Romanized North African author and wit Apuleius casually remarked:

> If you have said thirty years for ten, you might be considered to have erred through a gesture of counting: you should have opened those fingers in a circle. Since in truth you said forty, which more easily than the rest is shown with an open palm, this forty you enlarge by half; you cannot err by a gesture of the fingers, unless perhaps thirty years is calculated for Pudentilla by counting both consuls of the year.

What circle? What palm? What gesture of the fingers? *How* can the fingers be more reliable? Than what?

Fortunately, the Venerable Bede, writing in the north of England in the early eighth century C.E., in the middle of the Dark Ages, found it necessary to describe the Roman system of finger-counting in great detail for the benefit of large numbers of people who either never knew, or knew it very imperfectly (to their commercial disadvantage), or else were in danger of forgetting it altogether. Taken together with a few other medieval documents from distant parts of the Mediterranean world, Bede's expository *De loquela per gestum digitorum*, a section of his *De temporum ratione* (725 C.E.), is both a remarkable survival and an invaluable key to the ancient Roman counting system, which went a long way toward functioning as an effective system of accounting as well.

According to Bede, the Romans' system of counting with the fingers was built on the actions of both hands. "The hand ... was held upward, the palm flat [facing away from the body], the fingers together, except the thumb," which evidently stood slightly apart, not touching the index finger until it was syntactically required to do so. Thus configured, the following numbers were represented by positions adopted by the fingers of the left hand only:

1 = the little finger bent at the middle joint;
2 = the ring and little fingers bent at the middle joints;
3 = the middle, ring, and little fingers bent at the middle joints;
4 = the middle and ring fingers bent at the middle joints;
5 = the middle finger only bent at the middle joint;
6 = the ring finger bent at the middle joint;
7 = the little finger closed on the palm;
8 = the ring and little fingers closed on the palm;
9 = the middle, ring, and little fingers closed on the palm;
10 = the tip of the index finger touching the middle joint of the thumb (easily confused with 30 below; hence the significance of Apuleius's remark above);

11 to 19 = the actions denoting each numeral from 1 to 9 + that of 10;

20 = the thumb tucked between the index and middle fingers, so that the thumbnail touches the middle joint of the index finger;

21 to 29 = the actions denoting each numeral from 1 to 9 + that of 20;

30 = the tips of the thumb and index finger touching and forming a circle or ring (hence Apuleius above);

40 = the thumb and index finger standing erect and close together (which can be muddled with single-digit gestures; again see Apuleius)

50 = the thumb bent at both joints and held against the palm;

60 = the index finger closed over the thumb (as it is positioned for 50);

70 = the first joint of the index finger resting over the first joint of the thumb, which is held nearly straight;

80 = the tip of the index finger resting on the first joint of the thumb; and

90 = the thumb bent over the first joint of the index finger.

Bear in mind that hitherto the right hand has been entirely free. Now, the signs for 100, 200, 300, and so on were identical to those of 10, 20, 30, except that they were made by the fingers of the right hand, not the left; the right-handed signs for 1,000, 2,000, and 3,000 were likewise no different from 1, 2, and 3 on the left hand, except that they were deployed on the right. The round numbers of 10,000 and above were formed by placing the left hand flat on the chest, and by touching various other parts of the body, while 100,000 and upward were identically the same but represented by the action of the right hand. The system culminated with the sign for 1,000,000, which was made by clasping the hands and interlocking all ten fingers.

The beauty of this system was not so much that it was an effective sign language with which Romans could do business with one another and with non-Latin-speaking merchants from all corners of the Mediterranean, although that was sufficient to make it an indispensable part of daily life—no matter whether you were buying or selling livestock, slaves, bushels of grain, or bales of wool. Nor was its genius confined to the fact that you could easily make shorthand calculations anywhere, on docks and in the forum, at cattle sales, slave auctions, and dinner parties, but that these calculations were public, transparent, and instantly verifiable by anyone else who knew the system—in this case any Roman citizen with basic mathematical schooling. What lifted the Roman system of counting to a higher and even more ingenious level was that it provided the convenience, adaptability, and awesome potential of a complex system of computation as well.

The simple tasks of addition and subtraction were straightforward enough, and, again, could be followed with ease by anyone watching and verifying the process either for his own protection, or by a disengaged witness, tax collector, customs official, or notary. To add two numbers, one simply signed the first, then made the mental arithmetical calculation and reproduced the gesture corresponding with the correct sum. The process was cumulative; to add a further number to the sum of the first two, you proceeded to represent the gesture corresponding with the new total, and so on. Likewise, the task of subtraction merely threw the whole system into reverse. It was perfectly clear to anyone observing you carry out these separate procedures whether the job in hand was one of addition or subtraction.

Remarkably, at the end of the nineteenth century, related but very basic finger-signing systems of multiplication and division were observed and documented among Wallachian peasants of

southern Romania, who appear to have enjoyed an almost unbroken connection with the geographically corresponding Roman province of Dacia, just as old Serbian shepherds in the same
period were found to be able to recite chunks of Homer more
or less intact (usually less). Unwittingly, the Wallachians preserved a few of the methods of digital multiplication and division that were employed by the Romans throughout the empire.
The Wallachian system was evidently built on separate formulas applying to ascending groups or "cycles," consisting of five
numbers (one for each of the fingers of both hands). As the
mathematician Leon J. Richardson demonstrated in 1916, for
the numbers 6 to 10, the formula was evidently

$$10 \, (a + b) + cd$$

where a = the extended fingers of the right hand, one, two, three,
four, or five, denoting in each case a numerical value; b = likewise,
the extended fingers of the left hand; c = the closed fingers of the
right hand; and d = the closed fingers of the left hand.

The system is clunky, laborious even, but nevertheless ingenious. Suppose we do the multiplication 7 × 7. According to the
Wallachian system you hold up both hands, fists clenched, then
extend the right thumb and index finger (= 7), and extend the
left thumb and index finger (= 7); this combined gesture means
seven times seven. How many fingers are now extended? There
are four, and 4 × 10 = 40. How many fingers are closed? Three
on the right hand, and three on the left: 3 × 3 = 9. Therefore
7 × 7 = 49.

Consider now the multiplication 6 × 8. Hold up both hands,
fists clenched, then extend the right thumb (= 6), and extend
the left thumb and index and middle fingers (= 8); this means
six times eight. How many fingers are extended? There are four,
and 4 × 10 = 40. How many fingers are closed? Four on the

right hand, and two on the left: 4 × 2 = 8. Therefore 6 × 8 = 48. So far so good. But what about larger sums? The formulas that applied to rising increments of five numbers were

for the numbers 11 to 15: 15 $(a + b) + cd + 75$;
for the numbers 16 to 20: 20 $(a + b) + cd + 200$;
for the numbers 21 to 25: 25 $(a + b) + cd + 375$;
and for the numbers 26 to 30: 30 $(a + b) + cd + 600$,

where, just as before, a = the extended fingers of the right hand; b = the extended fingers of the left hand; c = the closed fingers of the right hand; and d = the closed fingers of the left hand. How then do we do the multiplication 12 × 13? Hold up both hands, fists clenched, then extend the right thumb and index finger (= 12), and extend the left thumb and index and middle fingers (= 13)—which means twelve times thirteen. Note that in each ascending cycle of five numbers the fingers correspond to a new set of numerical values, in this case the range from 11 to 15. You obviously needed to be very clear about which cycle you were using. How many fingers are now extended? There are five, and 5 × 15 = 75. How many fingers are folded over? Three on the right hand, and two on the left: 3 × 2 = 6. So, according to the formula, 75 + 6 + 75 = 156. Therefore, 12 × 13 = 156.

The drawback of this system of multiplication was that it required different formulas for successive groups of five numbers, and obviously also at the very least a working knowledge of the basic multiplication tables. Why not simply go ahead and do the mental arithmetic, and not bother with the fingers? But clearly this practice had the same crosslinguistic advantages of visibility and transparency among farmers, merchants, and tradesmen that made the Roman systems of digital addition and subtraction so useful. It worked, and worked moreover quite apart from whether or not you were functionally literate. Its greatest weakness was that the available parameters of calculation were severely limited—in these three instances to calculations consisting of 6, 7, 8, 9, or 10 × or ÷ 6, 7, 8, 9, or 10; 11, 12, 13, 14, or 15 × or ÷ 11, 12, 13, 14, or 15; and so on up the line, though it is not hard to see that in the nineteenth-century Wallachian village calculations relating to harvest days, viable fruit trees, egg-laying hens, poddy lambs, sows, children, and sacks of potatoes might be handled easily and often within the limitations imposed by each narrow cycle of numerals and their corresponding finger gestures.

In the ancient world, poor literacy, even illiteracy, was not necessarily the same thing as innumeracy—on the contrary—and in this enterprise the fingers evidently yielded an astonishingly sophisticated system of computation of which this Wallachian iteration was merely a dim shadow, much diminished by intervening centuries and geographical containment. And the lost prototype did not even require knots (as in pre-Columbian America), various types of abacus, or for the practitioner even good hearing or eyesight, although keeping a permanent record of numbers and calculations was obviously quite another matter. As we have already seen, the work of professional scribes was in this respect still an indispensable part of daily life.

The ubiquity of this Roman system of digital computation throws into splendid relief several commercial realities of daily life in the ancient world. Obviously, shaking hands on a business agreement arising from detailed haggling or negotiation was not merely apt, but a real, physical acknowledgment of the bona fide conclusion of a transaction for which the same hands strove to calculate and agree upon the fine detail. Payments in cash, moreover, mostly consisted of gold and silver coins, fairly often minted with a disembodied symbolic handclasp on the reverse, the thumbs interlocked but the fingers often extended,

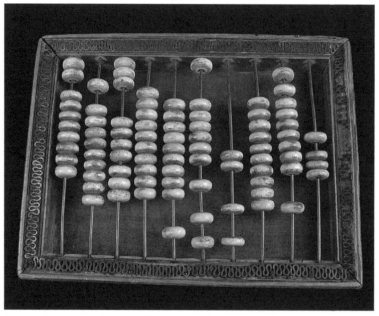

Knots, abacuses, and eventually more and more complex forms of notation superseded methods of calculation that were in many places practiced on the fingers alone. To skillful ancient Roman merchants, abacuses seemed especially redundant.

which as far as I can see does not necessarily relate to the value of the coin, but nevertheless brings to mind the basic conduct of the business of counting—counting goods as well as money—as much as it evokes the more familiar, indeed "higher" ideals of integrity and trust. That the Roman *digitus* should simultaneously function as a powerful rhetorical device, a form of measurement, and an instrument of calculation requires the modern mind to imagine a completely different and much more mathematically acute ancient Roman eye for number and proportion, extending from the jar of olive oil, through the contents of a basket, the capacity of the cargo hold of a trireme bringing valuable grain from the wealthy North African provinces, up to and even beyond the sophisticated vocabulary of architectural forms.

Long ago, Michael Baxandall demonstrated how similar techniques of purely visual estimation and mathematical awareness of the shape and volume of barrels, for example, provided Italian merchants of the Renaissance the powerful mental equipment with which to "read" paintings that in this context increasingly called upon some of these ancient Roman capacities for swift calculation, which of course we have now so willingly consigned to machines.

Above all, there is also in the ancient finger-counting system a solid link to the twelve tables of ancient Roman law. In a famous debate that took place in the reign of Antoninus Pius, and was witnessed and recorded in detail by Aulus Gellius, the second-century grammarian, author, and advocate (possibly of North African origin), the philosopher Favorinus and the jurist Sextus Caecilius Africanus locked horns over the question and theory of punishment, largely various harsh provisions of the twelve tables, which formed the basis of the criminal and civil law of ancient Rome. Of these, the third concerned debt and debtors, and toward the end of the debate, Favorinus attacked "the rule that permitted a plurality of creditors 'on the third market day' to cut up a debtor's body and divide it among themselves," in the absence of any satisfactory settlement or bailout, a ghastly retributive measure that Favorinus declared was as barbaric as it was useless as a form of compensation—very appealing as it may no doubt strike the victims of Ponzi schemes in our time. Africanus responded by tracing the history and development of this grotesque law, defending it with classical incoherence—if Aulus Gellius is to be believed—by asserting on the one hand that a sufficient number of debt-settling mechanisms existed on the preceding two market days, hitherto making it unnecessary for this ghastly punishment ever to be visited upon any Roman debtor; indeed, he was adamant that it had *never* occurred. On the other hand, it remained a vital deterrent for the negligent, fraudulent, or merely profligate. In other words, according to Africanus, though never used, this form of punishment was an absolutely necessary provision of Roman law. Naturally, the idea of tearing a debtor limb from limb and dividing the offending body parts among his creditors acquires an even greater chill when you contemplate the fact that those body parts included the digits directly responsible for making the disastrously over-reaching calculations that exposed him to this fate in the first place. And no doubt the grisly practices of mutilation and re-prisal that took place outside the law, and in many branches of organized crime still do—nowhere more conspicuously than by the Yakuza of Japan, who practice *yubitsume*, or the ritual punish-ment of finger-lopping—carried for the victim a far more seri-ous consequence than merely losing one or more lopped digits. In ancient Rome this form of reprisal literally put you out of business, and for good.

Money has now evolved into such complex and, for most of us, opaque forms that we can easily lose sight of the fact that its purpose, indeed its foundation, was to stand for a solid unit of real and reliable value that passed, and still passes, from hand to hand—in that rapidly declining number of situations where cash remains an acceptable form of payment. Ancient coins took the form they did for ease of handling, and portability. Indeed, the coin was to a very large extent built to meet the requirements of the index finger, thumb, and palm, and continues to meet them very effectively. Paper money emerged in China, and bills of exchange (the revolutionary *instrumentum ex causa cambii*) among European bankers and agents of the twelfth century, as separate solutions to the problem of adapting heavy pouches, bags, even whole chests full of coins, tokens, or ingots for essentially the same purpose, to be discreetly stored, carried, and exchanged for goods and services, always reflecting an agreed-upon and hopefully reliable system of common value.

However, the same virtues of portability and convenience that made the invention of money such an enduring success also made it especially vulnerable to thieves and forgers. Just as all labor prior to the industrial revolution was basically manual in character and scope—and the more remarkable for what marvels of agriculture, construction, and art could be achieved with the fingers of both hands, and the pooling of the resources of many working in unison—so, too, theft was a vast cottage industry requiring great skill and finesse, as anyone who has been the victim of an able pickpocket or cardsharp can vigorously attest.

Among the surviving records of the Old Bailey there are numerous cases in which, happily, persons guilty of "coining"— that is, manufacturing, disguising or doctoring, and putting into circulation counterfeit coins made from copper or base metal— were betrayed by their own fingers and thumbs. On July 8, 1696, for example, one David Venables was tried for coining when, through a peephole into a back room at the Bull Head Tavern in Cheapside, a witness observed him rubbing onto copper coins a toxic brew of what is described in the transcript of evidence as "feag." Although he managed to destroy the evidence by emptying a glass of wine into the gally-pot, and tossing it into the fireplace, Venables's fingers and thumbs were nevertheless observed to be badly discolored and obviously sore, so he was in no position to contest the accusation. In due course the jury found him guilty, and he was fined and pilloried.

A hundred years later, Sarah Willis and Ann Sydney were tried, convicted, and sentenced to death for doing essentially the same thing: coining—in this case "silvering" sixpences of base metal by using cream of tartar and other, more toxic ingredients—and in exactly the same way, despite their firm denials, the evidence of their fingers proved conclusive:

> WILLIS: As to the dirt upon my hands it was copperas [blue-green iron sulfate, $FeSO_4$] and logwood [*Haematoxylum campechianum*, a source of vegetable dye] that I had been dying a gown with, it came off directly with a little warm water and some soap . . .
>
> JURY [to ARMSTRONG, one of the arresting officers]: How were their nails?
>
> ARMSTRONG: They were quite yellow, and their fingers black almost all the way up with rubbing.
>
> JURY [to WRAY, another of the arresting officers]: Did you observe their nails?
>
> WRAY: Yes; they were very yellow, and the fingers black.
>
> JURY [to HARPER, yet another of the arresting officers]: Did you observe them?
>
> HARPER: Yes; they were exactly as they have been described, and they were so for two or three days.

By September 1806, the fruitfulness of the evidence of fingers and fingernails in cases of coining was so well established that, when appropriately tipped off by one of his paid informers, Edward Rogers and another officer entered the house of Thomas and Matilda Miller and arrested them. According to Rogers: "[We] instantly examined their fingers and thumbs, and on each of the prisoners we found them green and yellow; I took a pin and pricked from under their nails, and took out that which had a strong smell of aqua-fortis [nitric acid, HNO_3, another chemical routinely employed by coiners]."

In the long history of theft there are many byways of superstition, but none is so remarkable as the belief among professional thieves working in Flanders and many other parts of northern Europe up to the mid–nineteenth century that the severed fingers or whole hand of the cadaver of a convicted felon served as a charm for inducing or prolonging deep sleep among the residents of a house, for ease of unfettered breaking and entering. In some instances the fingers and thumb on such a "hand of glory," as it was known, were carefully lit like so many candles prior to gaining entry, and on those (many) occasions when the charm did not work, the culprits evidently left behind the ghastly relic. According to William Henderson, an inveterate collector of folklore—much of it admittedly invented for his benefit by mischievous country people who were simply amused by his credulity—a sorceress in the town of Alveringen insinuated the lopped finger of a thief onto the altar of the local church (in the guise of a sacred relic), let the priest say nine masses over it, and afterward used the charm to put people to sleep so she could steal their property unimpeded. The value of surviving accounts of these old superstitions is not so much that they existed at all, or that thieves persisted in responding to them, but that the magical properties sought by the light-fingered should have been found in the gruesomely harvested digits of a *failed* felon.

Naturally, in our time there are few if any such convenient sources of protection from forgers as telltale stains on their fingers, nor indeed the convenience of discovering among the possessions of a suspicious character a charm consisting of the severed fingers or hand of a thief—convicted or otherwise. Indeed, against the malicious peddlers of purely fictitious financial instruments, non-assets, and other forms of counterfeit that today lurk inside our irretrievably computerized financial systems, there is but little protection so far, and it is occasionally disheartening that these forms of more awesomely damaging white-collar crime are so much more difficult to prosecute than were the coiners of London, or the thieves of Flanders.

Of course these more current forms of theft still require manual dexterity, but, unlike those responsible for circulating bad coinage in Georgian England, the modern thief may avail himself of the anonymity of the modern office; steal huge sums of money without needing to break into and enter a house; and never for a moment raise suspicion as, with sly satisfaction, he attains his goal merely by depressing RETURN or ENTER on the keyboard of his computer. To some extent, successful fraud in early modern Europe depended upon scarcity or lack of infor-mation; today it relies upon a surfeit.

Even when conducted honestly, however, the enormous tide of modern retail business against which most of us now swim can present formidable obstacles to the happy conclusion of what ought to be swift and routine cash transactions. No doubt many other people have endured the maddening experience of be-ing unable to attract the attention of an overstretched salesper-son in a shop or department store, especially when that person seems unwilling or even unable to explain, say, the substantive differences between one expensive machine and another, or is for the time being delayed by a frozen or inert touch-screen cash register. Shopping for computers and mobile telephones are especially painful examples, above all when you have no inter-est in what an "Ultra fast Intel® CoreTM i7 processor" actually is, or what benefit might be derived from "Intel® Turbo Boost technology," or indeed if you are impervious to the charms of "tri-channel DDR3 memory." But the more trivial the product, the more maddening these situations can be, in which case it is sorely tempting to initiate a simple dialog along the following lines: "I have come into your shop. I have some money. I will give you some of that money in exchange for one of your products." Somehow it is rarely, if ever, as easy as that.

Certainly the advantage of carrying and using cash is that one is constantly made aware of what one is spending, and how often, whereas it may well prove to be one of the most serious weaknesses of the vast global economy that we have so deliberately built up that millions of people equipped with costly credit "facilities" may now dispose of large sums of borrowed money without much real awareness of what they are doing, or exactly how much money they are committing themselves eventually to pay back with substantial additional sums in interest. The woes of the present economy are the more desperate for our apparent inability to confront the interlocking problems of greed and hunger. The more we consume, the more we think we want, and indeed the more we want, the more our unreasonable appetites are whetted. Meanwhile, the poor get far, far poorer. As the eldest of my wise brothers has remarked to me on more than one occasion, in many places something as quotidian as coffee now comes in "tall" (the equivalent of what used to be "small"), *"grande," "venti," "doppio,"* and so on, where once it simply came in a "cup."

SIX

Gloves

Hull, in his *History of the Glove Trade*, says that Charles IV., King of Spain, was so much under the influence of any lady who wore white kid gloves, that the use of them at Court was strictly prohibited.

—Philip S. King, *Notes and Queries*, 1852

Over the past fifty years, nothing has disappeared so completely from the standard repertoire of personal accessories, worn or carried in many different forms at all times of day by men and women alike, as the glove. Hats, shoes, belts, spectacles, and most forms of clothing have changed utterly, but most (apart from nonbridal veils, separate stockings, girdles, and sock and other suspenders) remain widely available in some evolved form or another, and whereas gloves obviously still exist in places where they are needed for warmth or utility or protection in work or play, as a standard embellishment of the hand, worn incessantly as an indispensable ingredient of regular costume, most other gloves have simply evaporated.

In the nineteenth century, the wearing of gloves transcended most barriers of gender, class, profession, and nationality. It was simply taken for granted that all people who could afford them invariably wore or, at least, carried gloves almost wherever they went, even brides, who unbuttoned, rolled back, and tucked the lower, or "hand," portion of the left glove into the wrist, or "arm," part in order to receive the ring. Fashion writing in *The Queen* (from 1862 onward) and other mid- to late Victorian society papers is generally silent on the subject of gloves, for the simple reason that everybody had them, and usually chose from a relatively limited range of colors and styles. They are, however, omnipresent in stiff, wood-engraved illustrations, and while the constant oscillation of style in hats, silhouettes, ever new fabrics, pleating, "line," ribbons, varieties of lace, fur, and other types of elaboration was incessantly remarked upon, at inordinate length, the aesthetic aspect of gloves is rarely noted except in an industrial or trade context, as in the short-lived *Hosier and Glover*, "an illustrated monthly journal for hosiers, glovers, outfitters, umbrella and portmanteau manufacturers, hatters and clothiers."

There are exceptions to this general trend. At the beginning of the reign of Queen Victoria, the Parisian inventor P. F. Sole announced a new, ingenious, and conveniently nonspecific technique of cleaning dirty kid gloves of all colors "so as to look equal to new," a service he advertised regularly in *The Times* newspaper, for relatively high prices. Indeed, the persistent and publicly aired Victorian problem of how to keep them clean in what by any standard were public arenas of unimaginable filth is, beyond the default requirement of Victorian modesty, a partial explanation for why gloves were a daily necessity, and not merely an embellishment or affectation. For beyond the polished balustrade, knocker, or doorknob (in the case of well-maintained private premises) in nineteenth-century city streets and public buildings, uncovered fingers came into contact with any number of sources of grime that have now been largely suppressed by the liberal use of solvents. That we, the relatively recent descendants of habitual glove-wearers, powerfully emboldened by modern medicine, now choose to caress with uncovered hands the residues of so many powerful, dirt-obliterating chemicals is little short of an act of faith in a largely secular, postindustrial society that, given the high incidence of cancer, offers no guarantee that it is not fearfully misplaced. And we know the germs are still there. In fact, Victorian gloves were not free of health scares either, arising from the use of new synthetic chemical dyes. In the summer of 1878, for example, the "now fashionable 'bronze-green' silk gloves" caused widespread swelling and blisters on English hands, and the finger of blame was in this case directed toward the manufacturers, Dent, Allcroft and Co., who claimed somewhat injudiciously that male employees at the dye works that provided the color had for years had their hands "steeped in it for several hours each day," apparently without suffering "injurious effect upon the skin or general health." Not surprisingly, bronze-green gloves immediately went out of fashion.

In any case, nineteenth-century accounts of the British and American duties paid on imported gloves relate as much as £3,100 for 140,500 pairs of men's and women's leather and "habit" gloves and mitts, and were published annually in the press, because they bore upon the important and regularly recurring question as to the appropriate level of protection afforded to local manufacturers. The economic importance of the international glove trade—not by any means the least important stakeholder in the prolonged nineteenth- and early-twentieth-century debate about protection versus free trade—is an elementary demonstration of the ubiquity of the glove.

As with many other social conventions, glove-wearing was powerfully reinforced by the throne. For centuries, gloves formed part of coronation rites and regalia. In France the blessing and presentation of a pair of richly decorated gloves to the newly crowned monarch was held to be a symbol of the loyalty of his people. The emphasis was slightly different in England. Like many of her predecessors, at her coronation in Westminster

Abbey on June 2, 1953, Queen Elizabeth II put an embroidered ceremonial glove on her right hand immediately prior to receiving the scepter, both glove and scepter constituting powerful symbols of temporal authority, with more than a vague allusion also to priestly office. Royal and chivalrous glove-wearing (and gauntlet-throwing) habits of the Middle Ages extended back to the earliest centuries of Christianity, when the liturgical covering of hands was adapted from the practices of the imperial court of Byzantium, and rapidly became synonymous with high ecclesiastical standing. By a curious twist, the practice congealed around bishops, and thence made its way back into the habits of kings and princes, who were probably not aware that the Christian church and, before that, the Byzantine court ultimately inherited it from Roman emperors. In any case, royal glove-wearing appears to have solidified by the era of Charlemagne, when the Council of Aix (809 C.E.) made the decision to permit monks to wear only sheepskin gloves; those made from costlier skins were reserved for bishops and princes.

Quite apart from royal symbolism, by the complexity of their construction, through the Middle Ages and the Renaissance gloves were so costly and impressive that only bishops and princes or their most powerful supplicants could afford to buy them, and only those in unchallenged authority presumed actually to put them on. An exception was, of course, the knight's gauntlet, which, worn principally for protection, eventually acquired a higher political symbolism devolving from the crown, if not from the realpolitik of brute strength. Royal gloves were certainly widespread, even among the Vikings. King Magnus Barefoot (1073–1103) wore gloves of hartskin stitched with gold thread and lined with down, while in 1774 King Edward I "Longshanks" (1239–1307) was found to have been buried in Westminster Abbey wearing his. From the late fourteenth century onward, when King Henry IV (1367–1413) issued the first legal acknowledgment of the existence in England of glovers and an organized glove trade, patterns of distribution were obviously changing rapidly. To him has been attributed a famous remark to the effect that three countries were needed to make the finest gloves: Spain for good leather, France for tanning and cutting it, and England for the best sewing.

Clearly the finest examples of the craft, with many kinds of embellishment, were reserved for monarchs or queens consort until at least the second half of the sixteenth century, when Mary of Austria (1505–58), the sister of Emperor Charles V, bequeathed at least three hundred pairs. In France, according to Pierre de Bourdeille, abbé de Brantôme, Queen Catherine de Médicis (1519–89) "possessed the most beautiful hand ever seen," and made it known that she wore rich gloves because they actually enhanced the natural beauty of her hand, attracting "much attention and compliment." The trope of the beautiful hand, protected from work and sun, extends all the way back to Homer ("rosy-fingered dawn"), but there are relatively few examples before the seventeenth century of gloves being harnessed specifically as fascinators.

Queen Elizabeth I (1533–1603), meanwhile, evidently owned hundreds of pairs also, and throughout her reign indulged in sophisticated political gift-giving of gloves, not restricted to diplomacy. The queen presented a pair to Oxford University, which survives in the Ashmolean Museum. As C. Cody Collins remarks, either Elizabeth's gloves did not fit well, or her hands were oddly proportioned and extraordinarily large. Another pair survives in the Musée Carnavalet in Paris, "the middle finger . . . four and a half inches in length; the thumb fully five inches long; the palm has a width of three and one quarter inches."

The same canny mind-set that led Queen Catherine and Queen Elizabeth to exploit in this manner the political potential and symbolism of gloves as magnificent personal accessories, the gift of which implied the unusual honor of personal intimacy with the sovereign—the allegation that from time to time Catherine gave the sinister gift of *poisoned* gloves should be taken with a grain of salt, surely a politically expedient and probably sectarian lie, carefully disseminated—may also be traced to many other sixteenth-to-eighteenth-century courts, where gloves were highly visible, and glove symbolism laden with meaning.

Yet in this crucial stretch of two hundred years, glove-wearing habits gradually radiated from the court circle and penetrated more and more humbler households, wardrobes, and public spheres. They become highly visible in Spanish, Dutch, and Flemish paintings. They are no longer restricted to the great and the good, except in Van Dyck, many of whose nonroyal English sitters wear or dangle artfully a flamboyant glove, far more gentlemen than ladies, although there are a few exceptionally beautiful portraits of English ladies by Van Dyck in which a glove more than fulfills a frankly erotic function, none more so than the *Countess of Bedford* at Petworth, in which the subject exquisitely dangles her right glove, from the cuff. These are admittedly rare.

Indeed, it has been persuasively argued by Marieke de Winkel that by the mid–seventeenth century the currency of gloves was becoming rapidly devalued. She points out that one portrait painter in The Hague, Pieter Nason (1612–c. 1689), went as far as to omit gloves from a replica of his own portrait of the recently deceased but handsomely gloved Prince of Orange because he thought the attribute by then too "burgherlike." Diego Velázquez's *Lady with a Fan* (Wallace Collection), meanwhile, wears gloves that are slightly too large, the finger's ends loose and intriguingly floppy. And with characteristic brilliance Rembrandt raises the question whether his sitter for *Jan Six* (Amsterdam, Six Collection) is about to put the right glove on or take the left one off, while there can be no doubt that in portraying his right hand expensively gloved, Peter Paul Rubens was

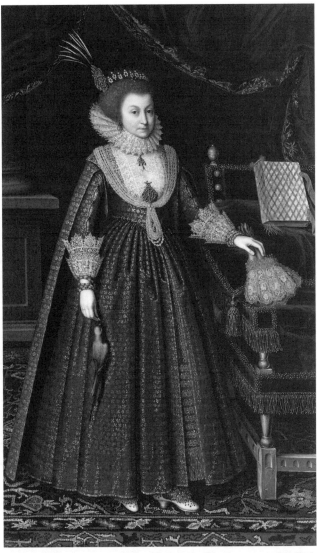

Paul van Somer was careful to document the Countess of Kellie's great wealth by means of carefully chosen jewels, items of furniture, and other accessories, of which perhaps the most extravagant is the pair of gloves upon which she rests her left hand.

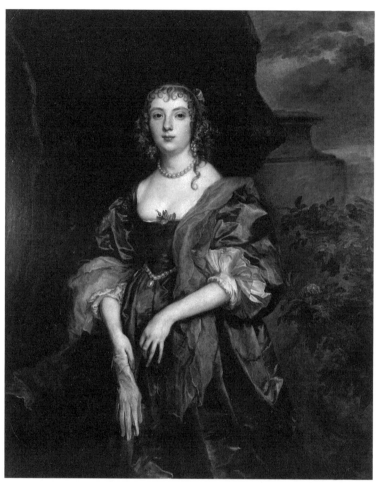

Anthony Van Dyck equips the Countess of Bedford with the dangling fascinator of a soft, pale fawn kid glove, a capricious amplification of the delicate ringlet that descends over her left shoulder.

affirming his own rank. In the mid–seventeenth century, glove-wearing habits were to some extent in transition, and by 1700 it seems to have been considered improper for Dutch and Flemish gentlemen to wear gloves except when riding.

By the mid–eighteenth century, the glove had become a standard prop in European portraits of relatively ordinary people who, though prosperous, did not necessarily have regular or indeed any contact with the court. In this context they generally make their appearance in outdoor or semipublic arenas in which gloves were generally worn, and are duly absent when domesticity is emphasized. Thus Sir Brooke Boothby, in Wright of Derby's delightfully recumbent open-air portrait of 1781, is sensibly and sensitively gloved, the seams deftly indicated, as well as the squashiness of the leather. But beyond this, the relaxed, somewhat fey gesture of Sir Brooke's right hand is surely meant to indicate not merely a snug fit, but comfort as well.

It may be a reflection of the intrinsically English love of animals and sport that, starting in the second half of the eighteenth century, portrait painters such as Wright seem to have earmarked the glove as an outdoor accessory. Certainly, a careful examination of the catalogues raisonnés of the work in portraiture of such different but great painters as Sir Joshua Reynolds, Sir Thomas Lawrence, and John Singer Sargent suggests that over 160 years gloves were consistently eschewed indoors for reasons that are not entirely clear to me. At the risk of laboring this point, of the approximately thirteen hundred portraits produced in Reynolds's studio, for example, I have identified only sixteen sitters who wear both gloves, and twenty-eight who wear one only—the far more appealing artistic contrivance because it naturally suggests that the sitter is either taking them off or putting them on, and therefore in the process of doing something. Of this latter figure, fifteen wear the glove on the left hand and use the same to grasp the other glove, the natural inclination of the

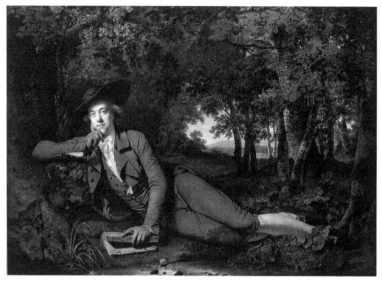

Wright of Derby understood the squashy, comfortable texture of the practical outdoor glove in his portrait of Sir Brooke Boothby. Even so, gloves are surprisingly rare in eighteenth-century English portraiture.

right-handed glove-wearer. If this habit is a reliable indication of right- or left-handedness, Reynolds took care to identify only eight left-handed glove-wearers—which seems proportionate—while there are only five instances of a sitter wearing one glove or the other without any trace of the matching glove. In another, very small cluster of portraits Reynolds took care to include a pair of gloves, in other words both held in the right or left hand—three and two cases, respectively—and only one in which there is a floppy pair of gloves draped nearby as a prop. In the vast majority of his portraits, such as that of the charismatic actress Mrs. Abington, Reynolds's sitters are winningly, sometimes in this case suggestively, even excitingly ungloved.

Lawrence, meanwhile, who clocked up about a thousand portraits, seems to have represented his sitters wearing both gloves only on four occasions, while eighteen of his subjects wear only one, and hold on to the other—in roughly the same proportion of right- and left-handers as we find in Reynolds. In Sargent's portrait production, however (about eight hundred works), we find only six wearers of both gloves, mostly military men, and a mere four wearers of the left or right one only, in which case the other glove is almost always missing. By contrast, however, Sargent makes rather more forthright use of pairs of gloves discarded here and there: more than twice as often as Lawrence did, and a good deal more inventively than Reynolds.

While the subjects of coronation portraits (on both sides of the English Channel) up to and including that of Emperor Napoleon by J.-A.-D. Ingres are invariably gloved—because it was (and in England remains) an essential part of the coronation rite—none of the members of the late-eighteenth-century Spanish royal family as portrayed by Francisco Goya wear gloves, which may or may not provide some support for William Hull's saucy claim, with which this chapter commenced, to the effect that Charles IV was unduly aroused by them. Actually, in Spain

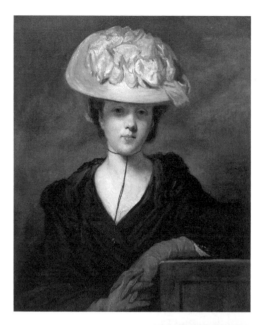

In Reynolds's brilliant portraits, directness of gaze may often be inflected by a subtle use of gesture. Miss Hickey's gloved hands naturally reinforce the shadow cast by her hat, while, ungloved, the actress Mrs. Abington touches her lower lip with the thumb of her left hand— a hint of provocation disguised as the gesture of an ingenue.

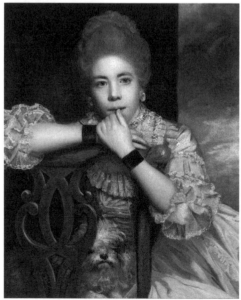

since the sixteenth century it was presumed that not to remove one's gloves "in company" was a sign of discourtesy. Even so, there are a few portraits by Goya of Spanish ladies in Charles's reign who wear long white gloves, most notably the heavily bejeweled and somewhat discomfited-looking Doña Francisca Vicenta Chollet y Caballero, who clutches a pug.

Responding to the first great wave of widespread public fascination arising from highly inventive new glove fashions—according to John Bell's English society journal *La Belle Assemblée*, white or pale-colored dresses should be accompanied by colorful gloves: yellow, jonquil, ruby, bright blue, or grass green—Regency and early- to mid-nineteenth-century portrait painters achieved new levels of subtlety in the representation of gloves, especially when worn, but also carried, draped over a chair, or discarded. On those few occasions when Lawrence included them, but far more often in portraits by Eugène Delacroix and Ingres, these artists variously captured the exact degree of stiffness that characterized the freshly laundered long white kid glove, ready for use, just as slightly earlier English painters, above all Wright of Derby and George Stubbs, understood with total precision the wear and tear to which ladies' and gentlemen's supple brown riding gloves were routinely exposed. Today we hardly recognize the visual contrast because we have forgotten what it feels like.

Upon the accession of Princess Alexandrina Victoria of Kent in 1837, the destitute glovers of Worcester, whose industry was apparently reduced to a state of ruin in the previous few years thanks to increasing competition from abroad, sought from the new, eighteen-year-old queen, whose heart, they prayed, was "as open as day to melting charity," an undertaking to do all in her power to alleviate their distress. In reply, Victoria assured the glovers of Worcester that from preference she "invariably uses Worcester gloves herself" and promised "those industrious but

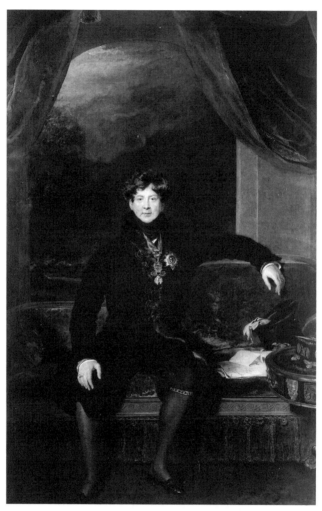

The Prince Regent was an insatiable consumer of gloves. In spring 1810 he ordered from Joseph Greves, "Hosier, Glover, and Elastic Brace Maker to the Royal Family," a dozen pairs of tan doe gloves; "white kid gloves with stiff top"; and six pairs of buff Lim[eric]k dress gloves." His hat and gloves are almost as prominent in Lawrence's great portrait as his splendid chestnut wig, the badge of the Order of the Golden Fleece, and his Garter star.

suffering people that no endeavor shall be wanting on her Majesty's part to impress the necessity of supporting every branch of national industry amongst all classes within her Majesty's influence." The queen also placed a large order.

Yet, apart from numerous advertisements for gloves, glovers, and glove shops, those few other contexts in which new gloves found their way into Victorian newspapers were generally lurid, relating to duels, thrashings, and other matters of honor to which a glove or pair of gloves was usually party. Fine kid gloves were mentioned very frequently as items stolen by petty thieves, or as useful clues in more serious criminal investigations. In 1838, for example, following the shocking bedroom murder in Lambeth of one Eliza Grimwood, *The Times* reported that a crucial piece of evidence recovered from the scene of the crime by Inspector Field of Scotland Yard was a pair of men's gloves, marked "S. K. R." These had been traced to the manufacturers' preferred glove-cleaning shop, where, by a stroke of good fortune, the suspect had left them to be cleaned not long before, and admitted wearing them when he took a friend of Miss Grimwood's to the Strand Theatre on the evening before the crime was discovered. It was further noted with barely concealed distaste that the gentleman's gloves were "lavender-colored."

Contrasting with the scarcity of nonlurid references in the press to new gloves, and presumably reflecting their ubiquity, there was in the nineteenth century a delightful spasm of antiquarian interest in the origins and history of gloves, not restricted to their distinguished royal, episcopal, or chivalrous contexts. Much of this was plainly eccentric. Scholarly clergy wondered whether the Book of Ruth or Psalm 108, where "the royal prophet declares, he will cast his *shoe* over Edom," did not in fact contain explicit references to the Israelites' taste for gloves. A Chaldean paraphrast apparently translated the ancient Hebrew word for shoe as "glove," an error that was cheerfully

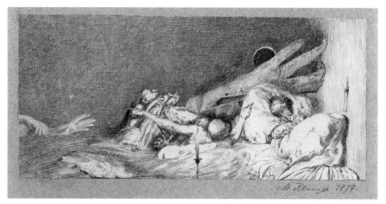

In Max Klinger's remarkable etching, the artist is overcome by a feverish dream in which a colossal unbuttoned glove stands in for his immoderate fantasies about the unattainable woman who evidently misplaced or lost it.

explained as persuasive evidence that Chaldeans liked to wear them. Egyptian mummies were discovered wearing striped linen ones, and in November 1922 the archaeologist Howard Carter found a neatly folded pair among the possessions of Pharaoh Tutankhamun. Some amusement arose from the ancient Greek view (in Xenophon) that the wearing of gloves against the cold was a laughable manifestation of the Persians' well-known effeminacy. On the other hand, it was carefully noted that Homer referred to Laërtes wearing gloves while gardening, which amounts to an essentially faithful but slightly overimaginative gloss on the *Odyssey*, 24:226–31.Varro thought that olives gathered by ungloved fingers were superior to the other sort, while a "celebrated" glutton in Athenaeus always wore gloves in the dining room so he could handle hotter meat than his fellow guests and thereby devour more, sooner. Pliny the Younger gave dictation to a scribe who prudently put on gloves after it got cold so he could keep writing. It was noted with interest, incidentally, that the Romans distinguished between fingerless mittens (*chirothocae*) and bona fide gloves (*manicae* or *digitalia*).

Renaissance gloves were evidently even more interesting to the Victorian mind than the antique or medieval, and in England the calendars of state papers (foreign and domestic) were scoured for references to diplomatic gifts of gloves such as have already been noted, as well as luxurious gloves perfumed with ambergris, musk, civet, or rose petals that were imported from Spain (Queen Mary). Not particularly busy Church of England rectors interested themselves in the identity of "persons to whom gloves were given at the consecration of Bishops" (King Charles I), and indeed occasions upon which gloves fulfilled all kinds of other functions, as precious gifts, love tokens, and "challenges of subjective belief, or evidences of objective truth"—for example, as a sign or voucher of entitlement to property, an early form of check or promissory note, legally redeemable.

Indeed, gloves long retained their ceremonial and commemorative functions. It was from time to time reported in the British law columns that a pair of white gloves had been presented to a judge or magistrate by the aldermen of certain towns and boroughs, an ancient and forlornly infrequent custom that indicated that there were, at that moment, happily no prisoners to be tried at the assizes. When in 1789, following King George III's recovery from his first critical attack of porphyria, Knowles the glover of 92 Fleet Street placed an advertisement in *The Times* headed "RESTORATION GLOVES," in which he respectfully informed "the Nobility and Gentry, that he has completed a large and elegant Assortment of GLOVES, in Honour of his MAJESTY's happy recovery. As the demand for the RESTORATION GLOVES must unavoidably be very great, the ornaments being so excellently adapted for the THANKSGIVING DAY...Ladies and Gentlemen will be early in their commands, to avoid disappointment."

This type of acknowledgment was not necessarily reserved for monarchs. At a ball held in his honor in Baltimore, Maryland, in December 1824, stooping to kiss one by one the hands of the ladies who were presented to him, General the Marquis de Lafayette, that great hero of the American Revolution, was shocked to find that the back of each lady's glove was decorated with a commemorative portrait of himself. Faced with the choice between fulfilling the obligation to go ahead and kiss hands, as was courteous and proper, or, from motives of equally justifiable public decorum, to refrain from kissing his own portrait, the general was temporarily impaled upon the horns of a dilemma. A pair of those commemorative gloves survives in the collection of the Smithsonian Institution in Washington, D.C. As recently as 1936, the Glovers' and the Gold and Silver Wire

Drawers' Companies in London presented a pair of ceremonial gauntlets to the Lord Mayor prior to an official visit to Canada, clearly expecting them to be worn.

Meanwhile, the importance of gloves to increasingly effete matters of honor stretched into the twentieth century. Reporting on a number of duels to be fought in France, on April 3, 1900, *The New York Times* reported that Baron Édouard de Rothschild had appointed Comte Louis de Turenne and M. O'Connor as seconds upon receiving a letter in which the irritable Comte de Lubersac threatened to throw his glove in Rothschild's face when or wherever they might happen to meet. This sort of ludicrous incident obviously stood in a long tradition, which flourished wherever codes of chivalrous conduct were upheld by people who regarded themselves as bona fide gentlemen, even in colonial Australia, where numerous duels were fought up to the end of the 1840s. However, even by then the tide of public opinion was turning against duels and horsewhippings. They were rightly thought barbaric. Occasionally people got killed, usually those who had no idea what to do with a pistol, and an intriguing subsidiary case against duels was made on the grounds that they were increasingly being fought between people who were obviously not gentlemen. The fact that dueling was everywhere illegal seems to have made little difference, so the matter of Rothschild versus Lubersac was not a particularly unusual or isolated incident. As with so many other residues of polite social observance, World War I put a stop to the practice forever.

Despite the tremendous degree of nineteenth-century interest in glove lore and, conspicuously, glove-wearing in church and at funerals (or not), the style and color of Victorian gloves were not often remarked upon in the press after the 1830s, when the celebrated Polish composer prompted a short-lived Parisian craze for white gloves "*à la Chopin*." All this changed in the Edwardian period. While servants, senior naval and military officers, judges, bishops, ambassadors, and high officials of every kind in many different jurisdictions continued to wear gloves, as it were, ex officio until well after the end of World War II—which goes a certain distance toward explaining their persistence as accessories in portraits by Sargent—in the first decade of the twentieth century there were signs that women of rank, and even certain professions and nations, were beginning to reject them. True, Pope Paul VI wore them at his coronation in 1963, and even more recently, in the South Pacific, a historically minded Anglican bishop gamely persisted in wearing liturgical gloves despite the tropical climate, but circa 1900 there were firm indications all over Europe that the days of the glove were digitally numbered.

In 1901, it was reported with surprise that, in the midst of the Dreyfus debacle—possibly in a vain attempt on the part of the minister of war, General Louis-Joseph-Nicolas André, to distract the public—the French army, whose 500,000 soldiers were each issued with two pairs of gloves a year (at a cost of 1.25 francs each), decided to cease the practice "from motives of economy." In Britain several decades earlier, it was questioned whether the only people who should wear gloves in the presence of royalty were serving military officers, and although there was genuine disagreement as to the correct form at Court or in church, one robust view expressed in the columns of *Notes and Queries* was that although gloves were indispensable items of Court apparel, they should nevertheless be removed when the sovereign was present. This almost certainly applied to gentlemen, not ladies, but neither was it the practice in earlier reigns, when gloves were routinely worn by courtiers, nor indeed in subsequent ones. By the time General André abolished gloves for the French army, officals of the Lord Chamberlain's department were issuing sharp instructions to British ladies and gentlemen: Gloves should invariably be worn to evening courts.

Beyond the tedious question of Court protocol, at the turn of the last century the more widespread tendency, noted with varying degrees of surprise in the social pages, was for working women to express growing impatience with the wearing of gloves, and women of fashion likewise. A gossipy complaint in *The New York Times* in 1903, to the effect that most gloves worn by women on public conveyances seemed on the whole tattier, shabbier, and dirtier than men's, drew the forthright response that "women wear their gloves much more than men, and besides it is awfully destructive to [gloved] fingertips to dig around in purses for change and samples, and to handle candy, to turn over books, and to examine dry goods." The same anonymous person thus defending the state of women's gloves further added that although they wore them less often, most men could afford to buy more and better pairs of gloves than most women, which was undoubtedly true—a statement that, for its date, is considerably more radical and far less self-evident than it might otherwise seem.

Slightly later, in the summer of 1907, it was reported from Rhode Island that the feminine fashion in Newport was to promenade ungloved, and that this seemed on the whole sensible, reflecting perhaps a wider trend in society—the "habit of going about with the 'arm part' of a long glove in place, and the hand thrust out of it, lending to the wrist a distressingly pachydermatous appearance," which was "unlovely and deplorable." The following summer at Ascot, "Queen Alexandra wore long gloves of pale biscuit-colored suede," contrasting pleasingly with what was described as "the inartistic white glove," which produced an unfortunate disjunction between dazzling white hands on black or dark fabrics, "never appealed to people of artistic taste," and merely owed its existence to the convenience of being able to wash them many times with bleach.

The next year (1909), American readers learned that "in London it is noticeable how many important brides have dispensed with gloves at their weddings... At the theater quite a number of ladies do not wear gloves, while others effect a great saving in their cleaning and glove bills by simply carrying them with their fans and gold purses." The ungloved hand, it was further noted, made it possible for women of rank to wear large solitaire diamond rings, which, with other types of finger ring, "look best on thin hands with bony fingers, the sunken places below the enlarged knuckles requiring to be filled out with rings of a showy type." The availability of consistently larger diamonds and other comparatively enormous gemstones flowing out of new mines in South Africa and other parts of the British Empire no doubt put considerable pressure on the glove, as well as the vogue for polished fingernails to which I shall turn in the next chapter.

In fact, twentieth-century English-language fashion journalism extending all the way up to the mid-1960s reveals an almost bizarre, whole-of-life determination to shore up the glove industry. Clearly this ran parallel with a growing trend of resistance to the wearing of them that, classwise, rose inexorably from below—a sobering reminder that the language of fashion and trendsetting may often depend for nourishment upon a root system that is either immovably pot-bound, or else clutching at the deep bedrock of unquestioning social conservatism. While few women old enough to remember wearing gloves as a matter of course would gladly resume the habit, one nevertheless wonders if in consigning gloves to the dustbin of history we have not dispensed with an accessory more than capable of at least exciting fascination: it is worth remembering that a really fine kid glove, with its rows of unthinkably minute stitches, is an object of exceptional beauty.

Because to some extent twentieth-century fashion designers, fashion writers, and photographers succeeded in creating precisely that: new and exciting expectations about gloves, as is evident from the array of frequently beautiful, occasionally strange effects designers aimed to achieve through an increasingly flamboyant range of styles, lengths, colors, skins, fabrics, types, varieties of stitching, number of buttons, clasps, and ornamentation. The sequence is breathtaking: in 1916, gloves with cuff bands of inch-wide diagonal stripes in black on white were recommended. Sixteen-button *mousquetaires* (originally popularized in about 1870 by Sarah Bernhardt, who was thought to have thin arms, lacking "volume"); black glacé kid, or blue gauntleting on white, were all de rigueur by 1921. White gloves, "fierce-looking and gauntleted," made an exciting return in 1922, apparently no longer considered inartistic, along with yellow on purple, or with embroidery "in some sour color."

Soft grays, tans, black and white, with scalloped edges, domino-dotted sawtooth cuffs, or ruffles proliferated in 1923. The following year the emphasis shifted to different sorts of skin: chamois, doe, cape, mocha, deer, buck, reindeer, antelope, suckling kids, and goat. The same year brought a slight "ruck in the wrist," and scarlet lining; "crushed" elbow-length gloves for daytime (a novelty); and gloves of beige, fawn, drab, pale ecru, cinnamon, or biscuit. According to *The Times*, at this date "the best English gloves have beautifully shaped fingers and thumbs," presumably tapering, while the body of the glove was either splayed—that is, gauntleted—or worn loose as a "sac" of between six and nine inches in length, depending on the sleeve. Circular cuffs with godets of gilt leather inset were observed in 1925, with riffs on white: ivory, oyster, champagne, beige, and, daringly, chartreuse.

Coinciding with but weirdly ignoring the Wall Street Crash, glove lengths apparently crept ever upward, and by the winter of 1929–30 wrinkled twelve- or sixteen-button models in pale pink, pale blue, and green, embroidered with pearls or silver, and worn with sleeveless dresses, caused general excitement, along with brilliant red, green, blue, rose, black and gold, powder pink, "nude," and white glacé kid. The deepening financial crisis apparently did nothing to dampen silk-lined mocha and antelope (1930), nor indeed to discourage the proliferation of amusing little bows nestling below the wrist or ring finger (1932). At the nadir of the Depression in 1933, chiffon and organdy, and plaid, spotted silk, and plain string for the country, were popular. In 1934, new *mousquetaires* of beige or prune-brown hogskin were back again, and also available in black, navy, brown, and, at 12s. 11d., "nigger," an unfortunate word chosen with care by Debenham and Freebody of Wigmore Street, London. By 1936, consumers were choosing among lettuce green, bottle green, pink-and-crimson, tan-and-rust, mauve-and-purple gloves, "van-dyked," frilled, even mouse-colored.

In 1939, the lowering clouds of war did not halt the production of violet-blue gloves with notes of black or, appropriately, thunder gray; mustard with brown or deep red; fir green with tan, or rust with petrol blue; forget-me-not blue, or camellia pink, bright emerald and cherry in the Directoire mode, all of which were prominent in Paris in June at the Comtesse de Beaumont's ball to mark the tercentenary of Racine. Somewhat shrill in their cheerfulness, the gloves of 1940 came in Goya yellow, sunset red, pig, seal, and peccary models. "American-Indian" fringes crept along the side seams and little finger, while various lacings offered cheeky notes on the back of the hand. These were thought to be "slimming."

With impressive resilience, gloves survived the dampening effect of World War II. At first, modest designs with downturned cuffs and lace details were the harbingers of prosperity in 1946. Then followed polka-dotted silk or "pique" sheaths with jersey palms for a better fit; crocheted gloves of flax thread; cocoa-colored double-woven cotton gloves by Shalimar; dark green "shorties"; and longer lengths—all in 1949, the same year in which it was afterward stated that "the growing trend toward longer length was of marked importance. Gloves were crushed in soft folds below sleeves rather than just meeting them. Even 'shorties' followed suit, rising a bit above the wrist. Fabric styles were noted for their chic, particularly those designed by Roger

Fare for Wear-Right with dashing sweep to their cuffs, many cut on a diagonal line and treated with contrasting color." Handsome eighteen-button satins for evening, meanwhile, were created by Viola Weinberger for the same season.

Pulses quickened in 1950 with the arrival of "citron," caramel, putty, orange, and the "Dot-Dash" by Van Raalte, "sprinkled with French knots (because you love nice things)." By 1954, gray-and-yellow was the craze. According to *Vogue*, "The glove news: not color in general but color in particular—shades of grey and yellow to glove a costume of almost *any* color in fashion. The lengths of gloves this year: ranging to eight button. The fit: satiny . . . Slate-grey glacé kidskin by Lilly Daché . . . Pearl-grey doeskin by Superb . . . Saffron French kidskin by Aris . . . Butter-yellow washable French doeskin . . . Smoke-grey washable French kidskin . . . Dove-grey washable French suède . . . Lemon French kidskin . . . Citron washable glacé kidskin."

In conformity with wider trends in fashion, particularly cinched waists, slimness was emphasized in 1956, as well as something *The New York Times* bafflingly described as "the new-to-the-finger-tips look of gloves," as well as "self-lacing," finger-length perforations for coolness, and "tapered rows of faggoting," all of which, it was claimed, accented and "slenderized" the fingers. In 1957, everything gave way to blue, blue, *blue*.

By now those branches of advertising that stressed the glamour of long evening gowns and sultry tobacco-smoking made ample use of gloves. Balancing a long white cigarette-holder between fingers sheathed in powder pink, elbow-length gloves, for example, a recumbent Marlene Dietrich purred: "I smoke a smooth cigarette—Lucky Strike!" Recommending the "tasty mildness, rich flavor, pleasant aroma" of Philip Morris, a peppier Lucille Ball was photographed holding a plump, unfiltered cigarette between the index and middle fingers of her right hand, snugly fitted in white pigskin. Purveyors of products as diverse as salted crackers, automobiles, beer, and soft furnishings regularly resorted to glove-wearing fashion models, the better to convey some sort of urbane respectability, or smartness.

And it continued. Immensely long, twenty-button glacé kid or skinny green gloves arrived in 1958, when the "fashion consultant" Mme. Monique de Nervo offered the following oracular advice to women in the pages of *The New York Times*: "'I would rather go without shoes than gloves'...When asked what she considers the accessory essentials of a wardrobe, Mme. De Nervo was quick to reply: 'Drawers full of gloves.'" Cheekier hints in the same year's *Vogue* presaged the not particularly well-hidden potential of Kayser's "Riot-Red" gloves: "Very likely should you try the fashion fun of wearing red gloves you'll find a gentleman's kiss placed firmly on your fingers too," while a decidedly more feline but no less ostentatious Dawnelle, Inc., suggested, "Handle him with gloves: Two on the aisle promise more magic than ever when the house lights dim on soft-spoken slim-sewn gloves of double-woven cotton, gently touched with trim." This collection sported ostensibly "Renaissance" colors, including Glitter, Lorraine, Monterey, Kingston, and Jewel Red.

New fabrics increasingly caused comment in the early 1960s, particularly the Kislav "washable doe-skin"—the name is a jaunty contraction of the French *qui se lave* (washable)—which was invented, patented, and successfully marketed abroad by the Buscarlet family in the French Pyrenees, whose chief tanner, it was grimly remembered, had been slain by the Nazis right in front of the factory.

By 1964, "stretch" models, or gloves with kick pleats, or daringly eliminated side seams, caused comment, while a note of desperation is increasingly apparent in the case of "Elayne," who, in *her* range of gloves that season for Bergdorf's and Saks, exploited butterflies, bees, black-eyed Susans, and "a pompom at the tip of an index finger, polka dots on the palm of the hand,

and black patent leather buttons around the thumb." A glove should not merely clothe the hand, she said. "It should carry fashion excitement."

This necessarily abbreviated sequence is astonishing for the sheer variety of possibilities presented each season mostly to women, but up to the 1950s to men also, thanks to the relentless "advertorial" of A. T. Gallico in the *Chicago Herald Tribune*, and many other, sadly anonymous generators of inventive, often hilarious glove copy. No doubt a good proportion of it suggests that midtwentieth-century glove manufacturers were fighting a losing battle to pique renewed interest, or at least maintain what had once been a universal habit, not helped by daunting competition from nail polish, hand cream, and associated manicure products, which, cheaper and easier to produce, went head to head with the glove and in any case were driven along more and more by canons of beauty rooted in cinema. The late Deborah Kerr might still wear gloves in *An Affair to Remember* (1957), but by 1968 the practice looked increasingly artificial, as for example when Faye Dunaway wore hats and long gloves in *The Thomas Crown Affair*—glamorous, maybe, but, on the whole, as contrived as that famously naughty game of chess. Meanwhile, buoyed by postwar prosperity, the increasingly adventurous travel, leisure, and holiday industries made the wearing of gloves more obviously inconvenient. Having reached its zenith in the mid-1950s and coinciding with the production of massive quantities of denim, the glove boom met its sudden demise in about 1969. People who for too many reasons may no longer be described as "stewardesses" stopped wearing gloves, a death knell.

Beyond its immense variety and unabashed charm, the persistent discussion of twentieth-century glove "modes," and the excitement engendered by different styles, lengths, even types of stitching—these often evoke worlds of total unreality, in which, for example, with feather-light touch smart women handled slip-

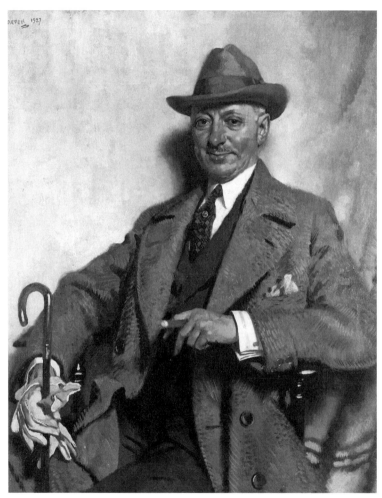

Sir William Orpen here accumulates an impressive tally of personal accessories belonging to his friend and fellow artist Jacob Epstein: tiepin, cuff links, hat, cane, and the pair of brightly colored hand-stitched gloves, one of which is removed for ease of cigar-smoking.

pery bone china; riffled through telephone directories; attached cigarettes to long holders, then lit them; wrote out checks; took charge of stately Afghans, or a couple of panting Pekingese; extracted small change, passports, theater tickets, or powder compacts from little handbags and pocketbooks with stiff clasps; manipulated binoculars and umbrellas at the races; ruminatively fastened strings of pearls and wound tiny wristwatches; balanced lightly on gloved fingertips small, freezing martini glasses; and caressed long-stemmed roses—performing each of these often fiddly tasks with blithe lack of effort.

To some extent, *The Queen* and *Vogue* and *Vanity Fair* and the fashion pages of *The New York Times* simply pretended that furry wet fingers, or gloves made grimy by rubbing maculated copper coins, or besmirched by ink stains or traces of marmalade or lipstick, or ruined by tobacco burns or soot, simply did not exist. Occasional glimpses of reality surfaced in the press, as when it was observed in New York that "generally, gloves should be removed before a woman smokes, eats, drinks, puts on make-up, or handles merchandise in a shop," in other words, before she performed what many men evidently regarded as a significant public act. Even long, elbow-length gloves, which were recommended for formal occasions such as dinners and dances, "should always be completely removed when a woman sits down to dinner." It is cold comfort, perhaps, that this sort of gratuitous advice generally stopped short of ruling on a woman's reading, writing, or working habits, in which case it was maybe presumed that she might, with luck, gloved or ungloved, work it out for herself.

Above all, and by contrast with the congruence of fashion and artistic representation up to World War I, as is obvious from this brief survey, the twentieth-century glove became gradually, then wholly, disengaged from larger developments in the fine arts, other than high-end textiles. Great twentieth-century portraits barely acknowledge their existence, and one seeks in vain the kind of relationship that clearly existed between the well-established glove-wearing habits of the nineteenth century and the sumptuous portrait practices of a Lawrence or an Ingres or a Winterhalter or even a Whistler, whose *Robert de Montesquiou* of 1891–92 (Frick Collection) ostentatiously wears white kid. Among artists of the first rank, the glove habit seems to have died with Edgar Degas and Henri de Toulouse-Lautrec and James McNeill Whistler and John Singer Sargent, Édouard Manet having largely dispensed with them long before.

Instead, commencing with Mme. Cézanne, proceeding onward through Dr. Gachet; Picasso's women (the tough, stubby hands of Gertrude Stein, the ferociously articulated fingers in *Guernica*); Matisse's lazy *odalisques*; Mme. Bonnard; the anxieties of Klimt, Schiele, Modigliani, Soutine, Beckmann, Grosz, and many other modern masters, one is hard-pressed to find a single portrait in which a glove is worn, or even suggested. One or two exist in the lonely diners of Edward Hopper, and Gilbert and George exchanged a rubber one in *The Singing Sculpture* (1971), but that is about all. Even Giovanni Boldini's sitters lack gloves, apart from his *Montesquiou* (1897), evidently a sitter who would not have been seen dead without them.

Beyond the self-fulfilling fantasies of commercial cinema, which have always acted as a sort of barometer of fashion, and outside the studios of society photographers, where occasionally gloves make a somewhat forlorn mid-century curtain call, the main currents of Western art, which in the course of the twentieth century pushed toward abstraction, evidently treated gloves with lofty disregard, preferring instead to take hands and fingers at face value, or to exploit the expressive potential of craggy knuckles, bony pallor, attenuated thumbs, or the flame red nails of Dora Maar (occasionally also bottle green), Picasso's sometime lover and muse. The painters of our era neither sought nor found any inspiration at all in lettuce green "vandyked" *mousquetaires*, and in that sense they were as prescient as earlier generations of artists who conformed to the glove-wearing habits of five centuries.

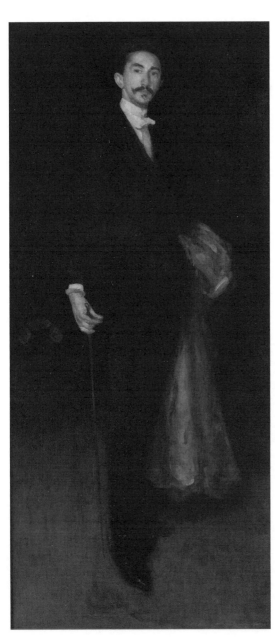

Whistler's Comte
de Montesquiou—
wearing white kid—
is, at least in this
respect, an exception
that proves the rule:
Increasingly, French
portrait painters of
the first rank began
to eschew gloves
in the third quarter
of the nineteenth
century.

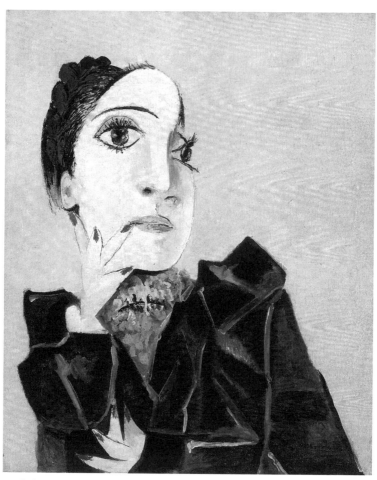

With her conspicuous bottle green fingernails, Picasso's Dora Maar is nec-essarily portrayed here as a fashion plate. Brightly colored nail polish was a fad that crash-landed in Paris during the 1920s.

SEVEN

Nail Polish

"Nail polish started just where most women's fashions start. I mean it started among women that most women wouldn't speak to. But it climbed, the way the other fashions do ...When depression struck America the women's finger-nails were the first things to go in the red."

— "The Major" to "The Post Impressionist," from an
interview in *The Washington Post*, August 2, 1934

In many respects the closing chapters of the history of gloves coincide with the rapid emergence of the care, shaping, polishing, tinting, painting, and enameling of the fingernails. By the mid- to late 1940s, while the glove still represented a degree of demonstrated chic, in many rapidly multiplying contexts an alternative chord was frequently struck, fortissimo, in the major key: that of bare hands with long, shapely fingers, and elegant nails, filed with precision into grapelike ovoids, and polished in saturated candy pink or, more often, glossy red. Increasingly, in billboard posters, magazines, and other illustrated papers women with slender fingers and unctuously tinted nails caress champagne bottles, carnations, and beach balls; apply Avon "skin freshener" to smooth white cheeks; laughingly dispense "chlorophyll" toothpaste; or toy with Soft Weve, "the newer, nicer kind of bathroom tissue." Carefully manicured index fingers and thumbs make fine adjustments to the temperature dial on a boxy Lady Sunbeam hair dryer. With feather-light, cherry red "fingertip touch," the wonders of "big-range cooking" are gleefully exploited in the larger kitchen.

Meanwhile, office machinery; a rapidly multiplying array of electrical goods (pressed upon middle-class shoppers as indispensable "domestic appliances," invariably equipped with many convenient buttons); lean, up-to-the-minute sofas; "pert and perky" foundation garments, aerodynamic brassieres, and one-piece swimming suits; seamless nylons; insecticides ("just press the button!"); even Coca-Cola (while for the time being demurer Pepsi women still wore gloves)—to say nothing of television sets, candy, canned and frozen food, and patio furniture—surviving advertisements for all these varied forms of postwar merchandise took advantage of the increasingly commonplace effect of moist dashes of intense color at the fingertips of beautiful women, most obviously in sunny or domestic situations where a degree of informality or practicality or undress made gloves plainly irrelevant.

There is a baffling instance of burlesque imagery in which a coy model poses nude but for a modest pair of moss green suede gloves and a matching beret, but this was an anomaly and thankfully never took hold—although I am told by a distinguished alumnus of Yale College that he finds this combination rather exciting. Even in the gleaming carbolic cleanliness of the operating theater, slim nurses in crisp green uniforms, masks for hygiene, and high-heeled shoes handle big stainless steel basins, amber bottles, and shiny oxygen cylinders with ungloved fingers, flawlessly manicured with fashionable tints, mostly crimson. Rubber was evidently at this date used only for tubes and hoses.

The English words *nail* and the compound *fingernail* are every bit as ancient as *finger* and *thumb*. In this sense, and perhaps not surprisingly, the direct ancestor of *nail*—essentially the same

word—rubs shoulders with the words for fish, cow, and dune in
Old Frisian, West Frisian, Middle Dutch, Old Saxon, Old High
German, and Middle Low German. In essentially the same form
it stubbornly picked its way into Old Icelandic, Old Swedish,
Old Danish, Old Welsh, and, with *bog*, into Old Irish. The antiquity and ubiquity of *nail* are hardly surprising, and because
it is so intrinsic an element of our finger we often forget how
remarkable and complex is its structure, and how much we depend upon it for the toughness and protection it affords each
fingertip. But what exactly is it?

Certainly the *Oxford English Dictionary* gives nothing away by
defining the nail as "a smooth horny plate overlying the upper
(dorsal) surface of the end of each finger and toe in humans and
most other primates," but this does not begin to sketch more than
merely what we see. In fact, most of the visible fingernail itself
consists of the "dead," or comparatively inert, gradually extending portion of what in the dermatological literature is rather
wanly described as "the nail plate," merely one part of the whole
package that emerges from the skin on the dorsal side of the terminal phalanx of each finger. That package is known to the professionals as "the nail unit" and, as a semiautonomous branch office
of the organ of the human skin, it is astonishing. The whole apparatus consists of (1) the nail plate and (2) the lateral and proximal
nail folds, known collectively as the *perionychium*, which hold the
nail plate in position around its outer, visible "edge," of which the
portion we usually call the cuticle, a thick rim of white keratinous
material, rejoices in the name of *epinychium*. Then come (3) the
"bed," upon which the nail rests, that is, underneath the nail
plate; (4) the *hyponychium*, which seals the distal end of the nail
to the end of the finger, where it usually protrudes—depending
on how long you let it grow—in other words, that tender spot
where we tend to get splinters while chopping wood, a place of
tear-jerking vulnerability, moreover, once much favored by the

very lowest of torturers; and (5) the matrix, the seat of the nail's growth, and to a large extent its health.

Now, the nail folds prudently keep hold of the plate by means of a narrow, colorless, but closely adhering *stratum corneum*, a thin layer of skin that grows out over the proximal end of the nail plate, and sheds itself as the nail gradually lengthens. This is the skin that manicurists attack with the aid of an orangewood stick, but might not so readily do if they were fully aware that, like the *hyponychium*, this *stratum corneum* is a protective barrier designed to protect the matrix from damage or infection. The so-called *lunulae*, or half-moons, of lighter hue that we see radiating from the cuticle are a product of the relatively tender and unformed keratinous substance that gradually hardens into the finished nail plate, in other words, the only outwardly visible sign in a normal fingernail of the ceaseless job of manufacturing that is achieved by the matrix, deep inside the finger not too far upstream from the tip.

Naturally, there is a wholly scarifying range of disorders and diseases that can overtake the fingernails (like everything else). Spoon-shaped nails, a condition known as *koilonychia*, is usually caused by iron deficiency. Then there are the consequences of what doctors refer to as "blunt trauma"—the accident with a hammer. This may cause bleeding under the nail plate, a "sub-ungual hematoma" and/or damage to the matrix, in which case the very toughness and protection afforded by the fingernail also prevents the little clot of blood from escaping. It forms a round or ovoid black spot under the nail, and if enough blood accumulates there considerable pressure builds and can cause much, much pain—so bad sometimes that the only solution is to release the clot through a tiny hole in the nail plate.

Infection is another problem. *Paronychia*, for example, is an inflammation of the periungual soft tissues, either arising from or developing in conjunction with yeast or bacterial infections.

There is swelling. There is pain, and there is pus. Another infection that can look just like a bacterial or fungal infection of this kind is in fact a virus, indeed the herpes simplex (type 1), a variety that carries the appalling name "herpetic whitlow." But what is so remarkable is how often these infections and related inflammatory conditions are a direct result of tampering with the cuticles and the nail folds in the course of a routine manicure. Likewise, the chemicals used in enamel and nail polish remover, cuticle softeners, primers, nail hardeners, and synthetic polishes themselves can generate all kinds of allergic and other reactions, the full range of which is enough to bring beadlets of perspiration to the brow, and a solemn promise forever to eschew color. The same chemicals that produce allergic reactions in the periungual soft tissues can also literally lift the whole nail off its bed, and regularly do. The abuse of certain hard drugs can achieve the same alarming, painful, and compromising disability.

However, what is most intriguing about the human fingernail is that it seems to have evolved naturally, along with the rest of the skin to which it is so closely related by kindred *and* affinity, to offer us the best we can hope for in terms of protection against germs and bacteria, at least on those occasions when they attempt to gain entry by that digital route. The nails seem very adept at sloughing germs, as much as the viscous coatings of brightly colored nail polish and other substances with which we now routinely coat them attract, harbor, and immure the same microscopic organisms. If there is one sure method of attracting to your fingers' ends the full and terrifying range of bacteria, grotesque flagella-dragging microbes—lounging in slimy contentment, treating your digits as an especially enjoyable mosh pit—in other words, of converting your fingernails from a healthy, borax-scrubbed shield of sanitation into the equivalent of a rubbish heap, it is to apply to them generous layers of synthetic polish. Into this congealing soup of cyanoacrylate glue, formaldehyde, thermoplastic, and epoxy resins, monomers, polymers, and other chemicals, even bits of nickel that flake off mixing beads in small bottles of nail polish, the microscopic zoo cheerfully migrates, while—and this irony is supreme—the various chemical disinfectants that are currently used to banish it from many manicure establishments, and incidentally to summon a mirage of clinical hygiene, can end up harming the very people who use them daily to protect their customers and themselves. Of the 224,792 cases of harmful exposure to cosmetics and "personal care" products reported in 2004 by the American Association of Poison Control Centers, nail care products accounted for no less than 12 percent. Doctors, nurses, phlebotomists, and indeed all other health-care workers are now routinely advised to keep their nails clipped short and not to polish them, especially not in germ-rich hospitals and clinics, and the only reasons I can think of for why this sound advice is not broadcast more widely to the rest of us is that the global cosmetics industry is very powerful; there are so many more serious things for us to worry about; people nevertheless seem to be prepared to take the risk; and, above all, it might make a considerable dent in the currently thriving specialist practice of dermatology.

One might be forgiven for concluding from the rich but cloying literature on the maintenance of beautiful fingernails toward the end of the nineteenth century that a firm and ancient distinction existed between texture or natural polish on one side and enhanced tints or colors on the other, but that distinction was largely one without a difference. Victorian fashion literature laid much emphasis on the care and maintenance of fingernails. It also marveled at the extremes to which French ladies of the ancien régime were prepared to go to protect their hands from the widening or blistering or discoloring or joint-hardening effects of carrying out troublesome manual tasks such as opening doors. That was what servants were for.

Victorian eyebrows were occasionally also raised by apparently anomalous instances of especially long fingernails such as the one so conspicuously mentioned in the exchange between Alceste and Célimène in act II, scene i, of Molière's *Le Misanthrope*:

> But tell me, at least, Madam, by what good fortune Clitandre has the happiness of pleasing you so mightily? Upon what basis of merit and sublime virtue do you ground the honor of your regard for him? Is it by the long nail on his little finger that he has acquired the esteem which you display for him?

Clearly seeking some rational context in which to interpret this strange attribute, which in the nineteenth century came to be regarded with extreme suspicion—as, in fact, it has long been recognized as an especially scarifying indicator of wickedness—particularly when sprouting from the male hand (even that of a Frenchman), one late Victorian glossist noted, "E. Fournier is quoted by Despois as conjecturing that this nail served to *scratch* at doors, as more polite than knocking." The intimacy of such an approach—the confidential mode of a lover seeking nocturnal entry to the lady's closet—was here discreetly overlooked, but even if the practice of scratching at doors was indeed regarded as more acceptable in France than the abrupt and peremptory knock, one must assume that either you had to scratch quite hard, or French domestic interiors were much quieter than ours. The practice may also have served to differentiate between people seeking entry, and servants.

Much Victorian ink, meanwhile, was spilled over the weighty problem of fat hands. According to *The Pall Mall Gazette*, "The hand with small nails buried in flesh is like a face with sightless eyes, or no eyes. The nearly nailless may be kind, useful people,

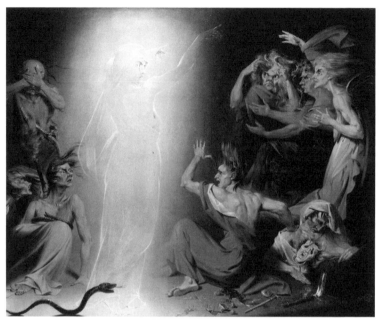

John Downman here deployed long, sharp, clawlike fingernails with particular menace as the ghost of Clytemnestra awakens the Furies. As an attribute of particular malevolence, fingernail talons persisted from the demons and monsters of Last Judgment imagery all the way down to Count Dracula, Freddy Krueger, and beyond.

but they discover no Utopias—they won't even tolerate ideality. The high things of holiness, of art, of human character, are not within their field of vision." More prosaically: "If your fingers are square or wide at the ends, you may narrow them a little by pinching and squeezing the tips. Needless to say you will not obtain the taper fingers you desire all at once, but in time you will become aware of a notable and pleasant change." Predictably, perhaps, a more robust approach to essentially the same problem in seventeenth-century Japan took the form of finger-compressing devices that were meant to force the fingers into a more satisfactorily slender shape. However, in Victorian England the nails were more important:

> Beautiful nails are looked upon as a precious gift. They should have a white crescent at the root, and they should be as rosy as the dawn. Pretty nails have been compared to the onyx by the poets—and, indeed, in Greek, *onyx* means nail... The women who have recourse to manicures will tell you that the ugliest nails can be improved by taking the trouble to push the hard skin that grows at the base: an operation which should never be done except after soaping the hands in warm water, and by means of an ivory or bone implement. The edges of the nail should also be filed in a gentle curve, following the outline of the finger-end. The surface of the nail, too, should be polished.

The art of the *manicure*, which before the twentieth century was the French word used to denote the practitioner and not the treatment, was mainly concerned with clipping and shaping the fingernails, tidying up their appearance, smoothing out their natural surface, and applying various fine powders and creams with which to buff them into a "natural" shine and rosy hue. Slightly abrasive tinted powders, when they were applied, cannot have made very much difference to the ultimate appearance of the carefully maintained fingernail, because most accounts of particular treatments speak quite specifically of these substances being rubbed, brushed, rubbed again, buffed, and then dusted or even rinsed off. This principle, far closer to shoe polish than nail polish, was not always understood, as for example when in 1893 a group of young ladies in Milwaukee, Wisconsin, were so fascinated by the attractive pinkness of the powder used by their *manicure* that they applied it liberally to their cheeks but found to their horror that it could not be removed. At best, Victorian and belle epoque nail color was designed to reinforce the natural skin tones, and not to supplant them with something new or radically different. According to the *Milwaukee Sentinel*, in 1883 an up-to-date *manicure*, apprised of all the latest developments of the art in Paris, could with leaden tact confide to a lady customer: "The nails are susceptible of an exquisite polish, and when symmetrical in form, free from all blemish, and reflecting a lustrous tint, can truly be admired. I am sure that if you had your own treated a short time, you would find them blessed with beauty you do not now dream they possess." In fact, the exemplary Victorian fingernail was for decades firmly defined by the term *filbert*. Curiously, a filbert is actually a hazelnut, and the hazelnut evidently acquired this other name from the same common source as the Norman patois phrase *noix de filbert*, apparently because by coincidence every year the fruit ripened at around the date of the Feast of St. Philibert (August 22, old style).

Leaving aside for now the baffling question as to why the comparatively lumpy hazelnut, and not, say, the sleeker, flatter almond, should provide a convenient metaphor for the ideal fingernail, "filbert nails" are nevertheless omnipresent in mid-to-late-nineteeth-century English novels and short stories, medical papers and textbooks, the fashion literature, and daily newspapers, extending well into the first decade of the twentieth century.

In a hugely popular story from 1845 entitled "The Lady Rohesia," the Reverend Richard Harris Barham observed that young Beatrice Grey, who attends upon her eponymous mistress's deathbed and arouses the premature interest of Sir Guy de Montgomeri, the master of the house, had "a pretty little hand, with long taper fingers and filbert-formed nails." Victorian fiction swarms with nearly identical assessments and terminology, not restricted to women. In *Framley Parsonage* (1860), Anthony Trollope gave us an intriguing introduction to the character of the Reverend Mark Robarts: "In person he was manly, tall, and fair-haired, with a square forehead, denoting intelligence rather than thought, with clear white hands, filbert nails, and a power of dressing himself in such a manner that no one should ever observe of him that his clothes were either good or bad, shabby or smart." In *The Woman's Kingdom: A Love Story* (1868) by Mrs. Craik, it is "the hand with its long fingers and delicate filbert nails—the true artist's hand" that leads Dr. Stedman to recognize in a desperately sick patient his ruined brother, Julius. And "His Princess," a racy story by the aptly named John Strange Winter, which is all about the doomed love affair between a noble lady and Dick Craddock, a handsome young cuirassier of middling birth, contains the following pungent but essentially unfortunate exchange between the two mismatched lovers:

"What a pity one cannot sell one's pedigree," she said, musingly.

"Is it long? What do you value it at?" he laughed.

"Why, where do you think those came from?" she asked, holding a row of filbert nails just in front of his nose.

"Came from? I should think you growed 'em," he replied, making an effort to kiss the fingers.

"'Growed 'em,' of course; but they don't grow by chance."

"No, perhaps not; the Greeks did not admire filbert nails," he said, coolly; "too near an approach to the claws of a beast, you know."

"I should have given the Greeks credit for more sense," remarked the Princess, superbly; "but since I live in the nineteenth century I am very glad to possess my filberts, without worrying about the ancient Greeks."

The extravagant assertion that filbert nails denoted high birth was actually supported by some antiquarians. Writing barely a year later in the *Journal of the British Archaeological Association*, Henry Syer Cuming asserted:

Long has existed and wide-spread is the belief that the form of our ungular defences proclaims the character and capacity, temperament and social rank, of individuals . . . Remnants of this ancient creed are still traceable in the popular notion that broad nails are indicative of plebeian origin, coarse vulgar mind, and unfeeling heart; that long or "filbert-nails" bespeak patrician ancestry, proud spirit, fervid imagination and refined taste; whilst sharp hooks are characteristic of all that is sordid, base, and brutal.

The accumulating picture of the filbert nail is fraught with inherent contradictions. According to Mrs. Leslie Stephen's rather depressing *Notes from Sick Rooms*, the British nurse "should be careful to keep her hands smooth and her nails short; the lovely filbert nails which are the pride of many are very literal 'thorns in the flesh' of the unlucky patient . . ." Evidently filberts were comparatively long, but not hooklike or sordid. They were certainly not broad, and, according to a notice in *Every Saturday: A Journal of Choice Reading*, the paragon of the mature woman "has still her white and shapely hands, with their pink filbert-like nails." So filberts were long, slender, *and* pink. Yet they gradually acquired even more abstract connotations. In 1911, a dedicated spiritualist and table-rapper noted:

> To me the most beautiful and interesting hands are the pure psychic and the dramatic—the former with its thin, narrow palm, slender, tapering fingers and filbert nails; the latter a model of symmetry and grace, with conical fingertips and filbert nails—indeed filbert nails are more or less confined to these two types; one seldom sees them in other hands. The Irish, French, Italians, Spanish, and Danes, being far more dramatic and psychic than the English, have far nicer hands, and for one set of filbert nails in London, we may count a dozen in Paris or Madrid.

To its length, slenderness, rosiness, the filbert nail now laid claim to prescience, drama, symmetry, and neatness as well. But in what sense did they relate to hazelnuts?

This question is surprisingly elusive. Victorian doctors were aware that convex nails, or at least nails that were too convex, constituted an unmistakable symptom of pathology, and they were right. When checking patients for *phthisis pulmonalis* (or "pulmonary consumption," as he called it), Dr. E. Harris Ruddock recommended checking the nails "to observe if they are curved downwards at their ends (filbert nails)." Yet traveling alongside this kind of observation was a powerful aesthetic that actually celebrated the convex nail—but surely not as convex, or incidentally as brown and as furrowed as a filbert. In a lecture he delivered in 1846 on diseases of the skin, Dr. James Startin stated:

> An examination of the nail on its convex surface exhibits a semilunar line, enclosing an area of paler colour than the rest of the nail; this is called the lunula, and is

held, when perfectly formed in a well-shaped nail, to
constitute a great beauty in these parts of the body, having the denomination of the *filbert nail.*

The implication here is that the shape evoked by the filbert
more properly approximates the line of the lunula than the
three-dimensional contour of the nail itself, which is reassur-
ing. Even so, public concern arising from the exact difference
between an unhealthy nail and a filbert was fairly widespread.
In 1883 a correspondent to *Judy, or, The London Serio-Comic Journal* inquired: "Are filbert nails more liable to crack than others?" Indeed, the tension between attractiveness on one side and
disorders attendant upon convex fingernails on the other was
from time to time implicitly acknowledged, as for example by
Dr. Charles Hilton Fagge, according to whom the "curved nails
(*ungues adunci*) of *phthisis* have been recognized from the time
of Hippocrates . . . [and are] quite distinct from the 'filbert' nail
of health." Rarely is it possible to see exactly how this is so, and
indeed the authors of the original article on "filbert" in the *Oxford English Dictionary* simply gave up: "'Filbert nails' are often
referred to as a beauty, but sometimes regarded as a symptom of
consumptive tendencies."

In fact, the correct answer descends to us from a brief and
actually much-plagiarized article entitled "The Management of
the Finger-Nails," by Lewis Durlacher, which first appeared in
1845 in *Chambers's Edinburgh Journal*—Scotland, as usual, providing a succinct and precise answer to a cloudy question emanat-
ing from England:

According to European fashion, they should be of an
oval figure, transparent, without specks or ridges of any
kind; the semilunar fold, or white half-circle, should be
fully developed, and the pellicle, or cuticle which forms

the configuration around the root of the nail, thin and well-defined, and, when properly arranged, should represent as nearly as possible the shape of a half-filbert.

If the Victorians ultimately tied themselves in knots over the precise qualities of the filbert nail, it is clear that the issue of greatest concern was that of shape, and not hue.

Vivid, saturated color did not crash-land in the field of French cosmetics before the early 1920s, but within a few years it achieved the dimensions of an enormous and plainly irreversible fad largely arising from the use of synthetic materials and solvents, beginning with durable (and highly toxic) fuselage paint for aircraft. In a relatively short period, the whole Victorian approach to fingernails was upended in the sense that shape conjoined with natural polish was entirely supplanted by shapes reinforced by synthetic polish. There was some resistance to these innovations on the predictable grounds of "taste," but the degree to which the old nail aesthetic was in free fall, especially as it began to take hold in America in the late 1920s, as usual after a delay of some years, merely serves to underline the irresistibility of colored polish. At first, there were objections to color—

> Every woman likes pink nails. It's a fad of course. Some seasons we have them almost red, and that's ugly. But pink nails have been thought beautiful from the time of the ancient Egyptians and no doubt the ancient Chinese, too, if we only happened to know about it. Probably this is because pink nails, like pink ears, indicate health and a good circulation.

—to color *and* texture—

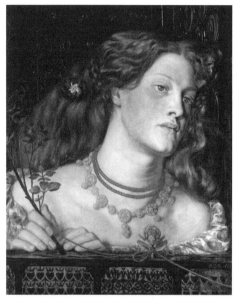

Images of "filbert nails" are as fugitive in Victorian art as they were omnipresent in nineteenth-century British journalism, fiction, and medical literature. Here, Rossetti's *Fair Rosamund* and Holman Hunt's portrait of Henry Wentworth Monk each seem to exhibit the several basic requirements of that now vanished fingernail aesthetic.

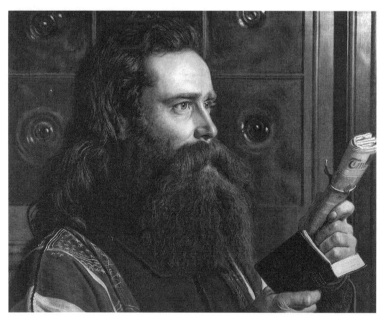

When in doubt as to what to answer when the beautiful manicurist inquires, "Will you have two coatings of liquid polish on your nails?" say "One will do."
That double charged shine is considered vulgar. Pink nails are in quite good form, but red is out in our best manicured circles. Of course, if you are one of the Daughter of the Nile type the ban may be lifted. But what modern American girl can look the Egyptian siren from earring to sandal and attend to her job? . . . The pointed finger tip, too, has lost vogue among the smartly manicured. The oval is preferred and the nails are permitted to grow longer than formerly. A small girl, however, should not try to adopt the Nita Naldi nail length. Proportion must be considered in even such a small detail as the length of the finger nail, but there is no question that a slightly plump hand can be given a finer line with a slight extension of the nail. A plump hand would not be able to take the extremely long finger nail test without its being made grotesque.

—to the risk to one's health—

There seems to be some doubt in the minds of a great many women as to whether liquid nail polish is in any way harmful or, at least, not so good for the nails as the powder or paste polish . . .

Many women write to me that they have used liquid nail polish and don't approve of it, because their nails come to have a purplish, brownish or bluish color. This, I must firmly reassert, is not the fault of the polish but is due to the carelessness of the user. Especially when one works in an office do such stains occur on the nails, due to carbon, ink, or pencil. That other crime laid at the door of liquid polish—opaque nails—is likewise due to negligence on the user's part, for nails that have been treated while damp will always look opaque.

—and, once these were navigated, to shape—

Finger nails tinted, enameled and polished to match one's pearl necklace is the latest fad among the fashionable women of London, a leading manicurist here disclosed yesterday. A new polish which gives all the luster and iridescence of pearls is being used and may be applied with a pink tinge to match pink pearls or with the pure crystalline sheen of the oyster pearl. Here, according to our authority is the latest rule for manicuring: "To be smart a woman must now wear her finger nails about a quarter of an inch long, the effect being to make the hand look as long as possible. The filbert nail is still the ideal to be aimed at, but it is no use putting a pointed nail on a stumpy hand. That would be about as ridiculous as a pierrot's hat on a little fat man."

—and even cost: "Extravagance in manicure will always be considered vulgar."

Certainly by 1929 the matter of synthetic varnish versus natural polish was triumphantly resolved in favor of modernity when it was reported in *The New York Times* that, of all people, Queen Mary had been observed buying liquid nail polish in Woolworth's while her husband, King George V, was convalescing from his serious illness at Bognor: "Queen Mary hesitated a long time over one of Woolworth's "forty-eight-inch, double graduated pearl necklaces," but passed them by in favor of toys, glass dishes, liquid nail polish, leatherette toilet cases, rubber sponges, and manicure sets."

Any and all attempts to mount a rearguard action against vivid color in the midst of the ensuing Great Depression seem from our vantage point especially forlorn, as for example when in 1934 Dr. Karl A. Menninger of Topeka, Kansas, presented his case to the American Psychiatric Association that "bobbed hair and tinted nails" were a form of self-mutilation no less harmful than the abnormal cutting off of an arm, or starving oneself to death. If Dr. Menninger had any point at all in respect to anorexia, he and other haphazardly energetic Cassandras could never compete with the steamroller of the J. Walter Thompson Advertising Company in its unstoppable campaign for Cutex—merely one of the growing number of hugely successful lines in cheap cosmetics.

In 1932, lecturing before the Royal Photographic Society in London, the fashionable portrait photographer Madame Yevonde welcomed the current enthusiasm for inventive color. In Paris now, she said, "women were tinting their hair pale mauve, green, or blue-white"—while their "passion for color has also spread to finger-nails." Madame Yevonde had even photographed women with "both red and bright-green toe-nails," though upon getting married one of her sitters confided to her that she had abandoned the habit of tinting her fingernails because her fussy new husband insisted that "it looked more natural thus when she played golf."

A few years later, despite the continuing enthusiasm for many different shades of saturated synthetic "nail polish which will not chip, peel, or fade," a lively exchange of letters to the editor of *The Times* in August 1937 revealed the existence in England of more sinister prejudices against wearing it, evidently not restricted to the better golf links. Apparently vacationing at 47 Augusta Gardens, Folkstone, George L. Massy wrote distastefully to the editor:

Sir:—I am credibly informed that the reason why some ladies stain their fingernails is in order to conceal the traces of black blood that otherwise would be discernible there. Perhaps the knowledge of this may induce ladies who have no black blood to refrain from an unsightly and unpleasing habit. It is understood that this practice arose in America, where the colour line is strictly drawn, and traces of black blood have to be concealed if possible. All the more reason for English ladies not to disfigure their nails.

Apparently not yet on vacation, R. Haslam Jackson, self-styled editor of the mysteriously fugitive trade paper *Perfumery and Toiletry*, of which there now appears to be no trace in any public library, responded testily from Arundel Street, W.C.2:

> Sir:—I am afraid your correspondent Mr. George L. Massy has not probed very deeply into the purposes of nail varnishing or its interesting history.
>
> Far from having originated in America to cover up evidences of "black blood" it was a common practice of the Chinese more than 3,000 years ago [*sic*]. The Mandarins went so far as to gild their nails as an indication of their exalted station. Later, Cleopatra improved on the practice, which already, for generations, had been followed by the Egyptian ladies. In Continental Europe and in this country women have stained or enameled their nails for centuries...The practice was discountenanced during the Cromwellian interregnum and revived at the Restoration; it lapsed again through the disapproval of Queen Victoria, and now, in conjunction with various treatments tending to improve the health and appearance of the nails, seems likely, in common with other beauty aids, to persist and to contribute to the prosperity of the ever-growing cosmetic industry.

The following morning, Michael Burn, the in-house *Times* correspondent, Nazi apologist, and sometime lover of the spy Guy Burgess—they cannot have talked very much about politics—observed that the ancient Chinese practice of gilding elite nails still existed in an evolved form, and much closer to home:

> ...There appeared recently at a fashionable French resort a woman, married to a foreigner of high birth, who had had the nails of both her hands enameled deep black, and engraved delicately with a small golden coronet. By these means [*sic*] she proclaimed to any who beheld her that she was a lady to her finger-tips.

The implication seems to be that, anticipating by fifty years the color preference of the international suburban Goth community, the surprising effect of black nails with gold coronets, while (at a stretch) in keeping with the fashionable setting, was more than vaguely questionable not merely on the grounds of entitlement—the highborn husband was, after all, foreign—but because women of rank hardly needed to identify themselves as such, nor so idiosyncratically, ostentatiously, even shrilly.

Ignoring these cowardly hints at counter-jumping vulgarity, but lacking the vigor one might have hoped for, the imaginatively racist claims of Mr. George L. Massy were nevertheless partly contradicted the following day by the young art historian Arnold Hyde:

> Sir:—I hardly think it can be maintained, as your correspondent suggests, that the habit of painting the fingernails was originally a device to conceal traces of black blood, nor that the practice arose in America.
> Lady Mary Wortley Montagu, writing from Adrianople [Edirne] in 1717, says:—

"... but it must be owned that every kind of beauty is more common here than it is with us. 'Tis surprising to see a young woman that is not very handsome. They have naturally the most beautiful complexion in the world, and generally large black eyes. I can assure you with great truth that the court of England (though I believe it the fairest in Christendom) does not contain so many beauties as are under our protection here. They generally shape their eyebrows, and both Greeks and Turks have the custom of putting round their eyes a black tincture, that, at a distance, or by candle-light, adds very much to the blackness of them. I fancy many of our ladies would be overjoyed to know this secret; but 'tis too visible by day. They dye their nails a rose colour; but, I own, I cannot enough accustom myself to this fashion, to find any beauty in it ..."

Although the exotic customs of the Porte were long associated with racial as well as religious difference, they were at least from the point of view of *The Times*, well clear of the United States of America, another prejudice that did not go unnoticed in New York City. A few days later, Harold Moody, the Jamaican-born athlete, doctor, and founder in 1931 of the London-based League of Coloured Peoples, chimed in with the following brief remark, which was no doubt constrained by the need to avoid dignifying the racist views of George L. Massy of Folkstone by actually engaging with them:

Sir:—Does not the custom of painted finger-nails originate from the fact of the "lighter races'" sense of the need for some "colour" in their make up? A European dare not appear on the stage without some "make up"—the effect would be too appalling. The "darker races" need no such "make up," although to my horror I observe how some of our beautiful girls are spoiling themselves by copying this horrible habit.

Apart from his pleasingly mordant point about the "appalling" effect of seeing a European onstage without makeup, Dr. Moody's brief letter succeeded only in suggesting that people of color would do better to avoid cosmetics entirely, a view that in 1937 was as plainly unreal as the cabaret star Josephine Baker was internationally famous. (She wore long, tinted nails, even in due course when wearing the uniform of a lieutenant in the French Women's Auxiliary Air Force.)

A week later, following several more batty communications addressed to Printing House Square from the library of the Athenaeum and elsewhere, the Anglo-Irishman Professor Thomas Bodkin, writing from the Barber Institute of Fine Arts at the University of Birmingham, contributed to this oddly all-male discussion a secondhand, putatively authoritative, but ridiculous coda with Belgian provenance in which matters of class in cinema were clumsily substituted for race:

Sir:—The interesting correspondence which has lately appeared in your columns on the subject of painted fingernails prompts me to submit the following extract which I have translated from a report of a lecture entitled *"Aberrations esthétiques de notre temps"* delivered a couple of years ago by Professor Hulin de Loo to the Class of Beaux-Arts at the Académie Royale de Belgique:—
"The mania of painting and varnishing the fingernails comes to us from America. Its origin is simple and quite comprehensible: the great majority of American women, even of those whose incomes would be considered lavish by us, are obliged, for want of servants, to do

their own cooking and household work. Such manual labours thicken the nails and destroy their transparence and natural polish; hence the recourse to coloured varnish. It is a fashion of unemployed cooks and chambermaids, and, naturally, has been propagated by the stars of Hollywood, many of whom have emerged from domestic service or factory employment. That it should be adopted among us in those too-quickly elevated classes which we owe to the effects of the War is understandable for the same reasons. But here the interests of commerce and fashion papers, who praise the practice and find great profit in it, are involved; and so our poor young well-bred women, even those endowed by nature with the great charm of pretty, polished, and transparent nails, which they should have no difficulty in tending and preserving, follow like the sheep of Panurge. Who would commit the crime of painting rosewood or of varnishing marble or onyx?"

The professor is a man so guarded in his statements that I feel sure his history of the origin of the practice is as sound as his objection to it.

It seems incredible not so much that Professors Bodkin and Hulin de Loo could concur that the gloriously colorful enameling of fingernails in the 1920s and 1930s was driven by black-and-white cinema, but that the habit could have been ascribed to the obscure origins, long-forgotten domestic obligations, putative shop-floor activities, or even the humbleness or poverty of a Mary Pickford, a Gloria Swanson, or a Pola Negri. Question marks might later hang over the origins of such screen sirens as Joan Crawford, and before too long an exclamation mark hoisted by Senator McCarthy over the head of that comic genius Judy Holliday, but in the 1930s nothing of the kind adhered to the reputation of Greta Garbo, for example, or that of the young Katharine Hepburn, or indeed socialites such as the limping Washington-based mining heiress, jewelry obsessive, and crank Evalyn Walsh McLean, proud owner of the fabled Hope Diamond, all of whom were by then frequently photographed in black-and-white wearing wine-dark nails, presumably but by no means certainly red.

In later code-observing cinema, there are some indications that painted nails still represented a hint of the demimonde, as for example in *Macao* (1952), in which "a man from nowhere" (Robert Mitchum) and "a woman with nowhere to go" (Jane Russell, with scarlet fingernails) "try to forget their pasts in exotic, exciting Macao, port of sin and shady dealings!" Likewise, in *The Unholy Wife* (1957), the late, glossily manicured Diana Dors, "half-angel, half-devil," turned the late Rod Steiger into "half-a-man" and "his peaceful valley into a seething volcano of passions that even murder could not stem!" True, in "Diamonds Are a Girl's Best Friend," one of the set pieces of Howard Hawks's astonishingly camp *Gentlemen Prefer Blondes* (1953), Marilyn Monroe wears extremely long pink gloves while being tossed here and there by men in tailcoats. But as regards the respectability of gloves, and every other aspect of that movie, there are in this sequence generous lashings of irony, something of a rarity in Hollywood. In the otherwise largely monochrome billboard advertisements for MGM's *Cat on a Hot Tin Roof* (1958) and *Butterfield 8* (1960), the colors of red and pink were in each case reserved for the lettering of the film's title phrase, and for Elizabeth Taylor's fingernails.

What is especially remarkable about the rapidly growing taste for nail polish in the twentieth century is the degree to which it, and various swiftly developing "tie-ins"—cuticle-softening nostrums; ever more complicated manicure sets; a torrent of hand creams, suiting a larger than necessary array of skin "types";

expensively perfumed "cleansers," as opposed to soap; not to mention the exponential increase in the number and variety of manicure establishments, from the demotic to the luxurious—ran neck and neck with the glove trade for at least fifty years. At times we may conclude that by the 1950s, when tan girls with shiny red fingernails hold bottles of Coca-Cola while Pepsi "refreshes without filling" soignée older women who wear narrow suits and peony gloves ("Men like her better"), this battle for market dominance was bitterer than it actually was.

In fact, these separate but related branches of the modern fashion industry stoked each other very effectively—just as, in the public sphere, women of studied elegance, or those aspiring to that costly standing, constantly took off their gloves, then put them back on again, more and more frequently navigating social situations both exquisitely gloved *and* immaculately manicured; modestly sheathed and excitingly lacquered, covering against both contingencies. There can be no more dramatic example than this intriguingly hand-in-glove state of affairs of what the French critic Guy Debord described as the highly effective creation in our time of "pseudo-needs," although I am reminded of a chilling remark made to me not long ago by a beaming consultant neurologist to the effect that imaginary symptoms are nevertheless by definition real.

To what extent did the nail polish phenomenon trickle down from the top, work its way up from below, or both—meeting in the middle? It seems that Mrs. Betty Ford was the first châtelaine of 1600 Pennsylvania Avenue permanently to discard gloves on state occasions, and I had thought that as the wife of an ambitious young congressman she might turn out to have been the first to wear color on her nails. However, this latter assumption turns out to be quite wrong because, according to her appointment books, Eleanor Roosevelt kept weekly appointments for hair and nails at Helen's Beauty Shop in Washington, and surprisingly often

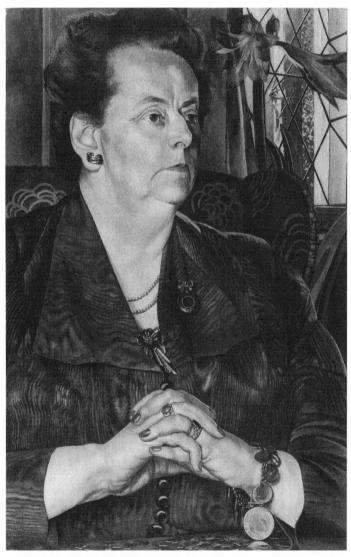

In Stanley Spencer's portrait, the formidable justice of the peace and lady mayoress Mrs. Frank demonstrates the ubiquity of glossy nail polish among middle-class wearers by the end of the 1940s, as well as the commercially manufactured jigsaw puzzle.

in Manhattan at Arnold Constable's on Fifth Avenue at Fortieth Street, generally on a Friday. Earlier I had presumed that photographs of Mrs. Roosevelt were merely fanciful as regards tinted fingernails, or doctored, but it seems that the First Lady did indeed indulge a pronounced taste for bright color, as indeed did Queen Elizabeth, the Queen Mother.

Twenty years ago the international cosmetics business was worth approximately $20 billion worldwide. In 2006 it was worth $250 billion. Even adjusting for the declining value of the dollar, this rate of growth seems to me astonishing, and nail polish and related products—which now include fake nails, ground coats, top coats, stenciled and other decorations, glitter, frosting, and so on—account for a significant proportion of that huge figure, while the constantly growing number of available brands, colors, and textures employ ever more improbable names. "Innocent Nude," "Pink Passion," "Peach Lover," "I'm Not Really a Waitress," "Catherine the Grape," "Melon of Troy," "Vendetta," and "Vixen" are by no means unusual, as any seasoned shopper will attest.

Likewise, as is demonstrated by the still-accelerating sales of little bottles of nail polish in hundreds of subtly different shades (and almost as many little bottles of nail polish remover)—never to forget the rows and rows of pairs of gloves that once neatly lined the downstairs counters of B. Altman and Company, and Macy's, and Lord and Taylor, and Selfridge's, and Galeries Lafayette, and so many other department stores—the truly sinister thing about "pseudo-needs" is how easily they turn into obviously real ones: pressing, nearly universal, and apparently insatiable, reaching all the way down to our fingers' ends.

EIGHT

The Finger of Play

I rose up to open to my beloved;
and my hands dropped with myrrh,
and my fingers with sweet smelling myrrh,
upon the handles of the lock.

—Song of Solomon 5:5

Bowlers with plenty of finger-spin are most likely to take wickets on
the mat. —*Westminster Gazette*, July 1, 1905

With his long hair and comfortable white shirt with loose
sleeves, the English schoolboy Richard Heber (1773–
1833), portrayed in 1782 by the American expatriate John
Singleton Copley, exhibits all the informality and naturalness
that were such desirable qualities in portraits of Georgian children, while the paraphernalia of the quintessentially English game
of cricket allude to the manly sports in general. Looking boldly
toward an unseen opponent, leaning on his bat and holding the
ball—which, according to an old museum wall label, means essentially "that play cannot commence until he chooses," though
it seems more likely to me that his ad hoc arrangement of stumps
and bail have just now been struck and that in the absence of a
wicket-keeper, he is about to return the ball to the victorious

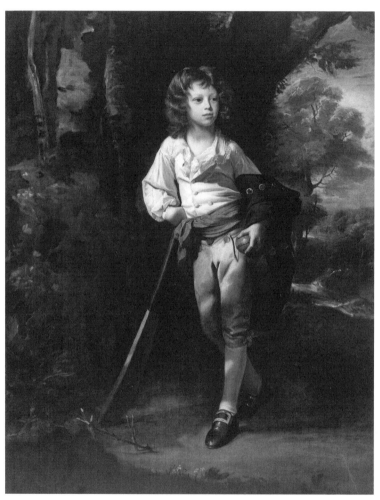

In John Singleton Copley's portrait, the English schoolboy Richard Heber leans on his cricket bat and holds the ball, prior to the recommencement of play.

bowler—Richard Heber nevertheless strikes an authoritative pose: proud, certainly, if momentarily chastened.

In America cricket tends to be obscure and mysterious, and this makes it possible for me to conceal my almost total ignorance of the game. I derive particular amusement from reinventing myself here as a cricket aficionado, something that generates immoderate laughter in my more knowledgeable Australian nieces and nephews. For example, I can explain the tapering, rounded shape of the cricket bat that was standard in mid- to late-eighteenth-century England. I speak with authority about the gradual flattening of the bat, the squaring off in the front, back, sides, and "shoulder" during the Regency and early to mid-Victorian periods. With luck and an effort to retrieve childhood memory I can explain how the boy in the painting might hold his bat absolutely correctly with both hands, or in later innings bowl the ball—maybe even with spin.

Nowadays the standard red cricket ball is subject to precise specifications, under the fifth Law of Cricket. "The ball, when new, shall weigh not less than 5½ ounces, nor more than 5¾ ounces, and shall measure not less than 8¹³⁄₁₆ inches, nor more than 9 inches in circumference." Compared with a Major League baseball, which ought to be 9 to 9¼ inches in circumference, and weigh between 5 and 5¼ ounces, the cricket ball is smaller, harder, and heavier, and causes more damage to the shins, yet judging from Copley's portrait the dimensions and structure of the cricket ball have not changed substantially in the past two hundred years. It was, of course, like most balls of its type, originally designed to fit snugly into the hand of a bowler, and in due course its compactness made it an ideal vehicle for various types of spin that bowlers (the equivalent of pitchers) artfully set in train with the relevant set of fingers, the better to provide a robust contest against the opposing batsmen (batters). The hardness of the ball is of course designed to withstand the fullest measure of force

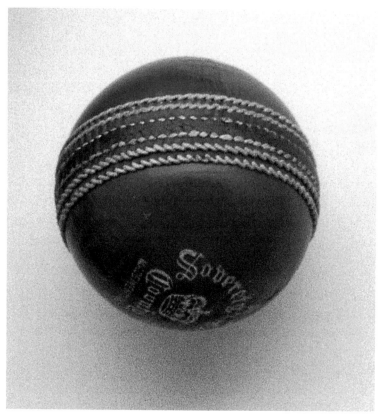

A standard Readers Sovereign Special County "A" cricket ball. Among the carefully differentiated and highly specialist types of bowling in cricket, "finger spin" is perhaps the most devious, and deadly.

that the prehensile digits bring to the task of bowling with or without spin, and catching it.

In the glorious history of the international cricket competition between England and Australia, styles of bowling have from time to time created enormous controversy, as for example in the so-called bodyline series beginning in November 1930, when in desperation to gain some purchase against dominant Australian batsmen (batters), English bowlers (pitchers) radically altered their bowling style, and by very accurately aiming the ball at the head or body of their opponent temporarily gained the upper hand. This was an extreme development, a highly aggressive variation of what B. J. T. Bosanquet of Oxford and Middlesex achieved for England in about 1900 by inventing a thing called a "googly," "wrong 'un," or eponymous "Bosie," as it became known in Australia. In technical terms, this was an "off-break" style of bowling the cricket ball, "delivered with a leg-break action from the back, rather than from the front of the hand. Bringing the ball over from a great height [he was six feet tall, and unlike baseballs cricket balls are bowled over the head, at the conclusion of a running start of varying distances] Bosanquet mystified the best Australian batsmen with its flight and uncertain break." He developed this method of bowling—or type of "ball"—by "playing billiard fives or 'twisty grab' and experimenting with bouncing a tennis ball on a table so that his opponent seated at the other end of the table could not catch it. 'It was not unfair, only immoral,' he said of his 'Bosie.'"

In cricket the finger also has vital demonstrative function, because under the Third Law, which concerns "The Umpires," the universal and time-honored convention by which a batsman is judged to have been dismissed—for whatever reason—is when the umpire, that white-coated sage standing not too far from the wicket, raises his index finger over his head. The sources are unclear, but received opinion appears to be that the origin of this unmistakable gesture was merely as a direction toward the place where the batsman ought now to make his way without further ado, namely the pavilion, "there being no basis upon which he should remain any longer at the crease"—which is the equivalent of the batter's box in baseball. Formerly, most umpires simply held their index finger aloft, in conformity with the practice as laid down by the Marylebone Cricket Club, but what was once a common usage has (no doubt encouraged in this direction by the influence of the close-up shot for television) gradually become prone to distinctive variations, the gradual adoption of a carefully differentiated, occasionally amusing personal style by which certain umpires claim their right to deliver the fateful verdict. It has also gradually been anticipated, preempted, and even at times supplanted by the successful bowler's increasingly triumphalist determination to decorate his dismissals with an aptly worded insult or curse, so that the broken batsman must now depart from the crease not merely dispatched by the umpire's finger of authority, but further chastened by rude remarks as well. No doubt this was what the late prime minister Sir Robert Gordon Menzies, K.T., C.H., Q.C., was referring to when he spoke of "the juicy humanity of cricketers."

In a fundamental sense the purpose of games, of play, is not merely to provide children with the exercise they need to develop physically, but with bat, ball, or whatever else, to hone the skills of hand and eye. These were never skills in which I showed any aptitude at all, and no doubt many children continue to suffer as a consequence of poor coordination, being rather slow, maybe even not remotely interested, or plain bad at catching balls or throwing them in predictable directions. Yet for millions of children all over the world the skills of balance and coordination, of teamwork, the nimble throw, the backhand volley, the true aim, lightning reflexes, together with the hard-fought points thus accumulated in competition, present an invaluable path of development, and inspire a sort of love that extends far beyond the years of adolescence—duly propelling adults onto the golf links, and into many other sporting arenas for the pure pleasure of practicing and maintaining for as long as possible those same skills, or seeing them displayed by a tiny elite who bring them to the level of near perfection. In so many respects, while it is conducted with various degrees of leisure, seriousness, professionalism, or fun, sport is in larger cultural terms quite obviously far more than merely a game.

It is no accident that the same English verb that we apply to sport we apply also to music, theater, and love. Music is *played*, and in this context *to finger something* in strictly instrumental terms means of course to adopt the correct arrangement of the fingers (for ease, or precision, or correctness of notation and pitch). In the history of music, "authentic fingering" is obviously of much interest to the musicologist as well as to the modern performer, but as it is prescribed in scores, and set down as helpfully as possible by composers, the original fingering for strings especially can collide unhelpfully with the musical instruments as they have gradually evolved, creating problems of interpretation. Does the modern performer follow the composer's instructions to the letter, or seek from the musical context a more convenient, fluid, or satisfactory means by which to express the principal idea that the fingering instructions were originally intended to facilitate?

The problem has occasionally come to light in the chamber music of Haydn, but it is in the fascinating evolution of wind instruments that surviving fingering charts themselves provide intriguing evidence for just how much those instruments have changed in the past three centuries. Through the eighteenth century, for example, a wide variety of fingering instructions were published relating to no fewer than five different types of clarinet with from as few as two to up to seven keys. Obviously

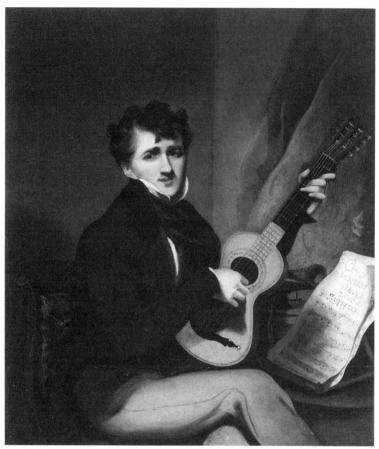

Many specialized skills of manual dexterity have vanished from modern life in the West, where once the purely domestic accomplishments of art and music-making were essential components of the game of love. George Chinnery's sensitive young man is playing on his guitar a new French love song.

the technique of playing each varied considerably, and had to be mastered in turn by the specialist pupil or professional player as each model was developed, embraced, and absorbed into the fledgling orchestra. By contrast, in the same period fingering instructions for the oboe tended to be standard wherever the oboe was played, but evolved quite rapidly to accommodate technical innovation, improved facility and speed, and also musical taste.

In these instances, and that of the bassoon also, the picture is further complicated by the activities spread across wide geographical distances of sometimes only a handful of maker-players, the needs and expanding technical requirements of player-performers, and the gradual rise and consolidation of the governing role of composer. But the larger point is, of course, that on keyboard, string, hole, or key, the finger and its capacity to convert musical intelligence into sounds produced by otherwise inanimate objects—often with infinitesimal degrees of nuance, pressure, precision, and touch—attain for us the deep and time-dependent experience of musical sensation. It is yet another instance of the constituent parts of what Raymond Tallis aptly describes as "the tool of tools," the human hand, sailing intricately and spectacularly over the high hurdles of art.

Not everyone is good at throwing a ball, and comparatively few people ever master the violin, oboe, or piano, but almost everybody has at some point experienced the ecstatic sensuality of touch, and imparted it zestfully with fingers that stroke or fondle, or merely intertwine through holding hands. It is one of the regularly recurring themes of this book, but too often (as we shall see) dragged into the sphere of violence or obscenity. In a thoroughly stimulating section of The Book of Skin, Steven Connor points to the importance to intimate human experience of our fingers, and not merely as objects of adornment or sources of accurate information. When we itch, then scratch, he points out, we use our fingers and more specifically our fingernails as a

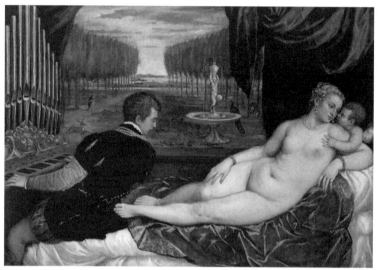

The explicitly erotic prompts of fingering the keyboard and thereby activating organ pipes may strike us as almost comically blunt, but for Titian in this and in many other versions of similar voluptuously nude subject paintings, secular music-making and lovemaking were powerfully intertwined.

tool. "Though they are made of the same substance—keratin—as the top layer of the skin [but rather differently configured], they function as something we use on ourselves." In other words, when we scratch we borrow our nails from the world around us, as it were, instead of treating them in that instant as a part of our own body. And in scratching ourselves we derive the delicious sensation of responding directly to the itch. In some vague but deeply rooted sense they also remind us by their protective function, and the fact that they grow quite rapidly out of our fingers' ends, of comparably "encrusted or encysted" bodily phenomena in the animal kingdom, from horns and antlers all the way down to the tough shells of beetles and crustaceans. Incidentally, everything with a pulse scratches.

As well, the simple, hopefully private, and above all civilized action of trimming our fingernails can, for at least one left-handed French philosopher, function as a symbol or metaphor of what Connor describes as "the contingency of the soul." In other words, the left-hand "subject," armed with the nail clippers, "works on the right hand object. The left hand participates in the 'I,' suffused with subjectivity; the right hand is of the world." For the time being, if for no other reason than the aesthetic, one surely hopes that that fingernail forms the comparatively disengaged object of rapt ministration.

The same cannot possibly be said of the finger as a shrewd but freewheeling participant in the game of love, no matter how innocent on one side, or ecstatically sexual on the other. It is the wholly subjective agent of erotic stimulus, the first toy with which we derive sexual pleasure from the discovery and exploration of our own bodies. It reaches out before we kiss and (with luck) spans the terrifying gap in distance between two lovers, and may either bring about the sudden collapse of that spatial distance or else recoil in horror if the overture is rejected. It lets us tickle, and responds with vigor if we happen to be ticklish. It

gauges warmth, and imparts warmth—often in such equal measure that, when your fingers are for a while intertwined with
a set belonging to someone else, you may feel hard-pressed to distinguish between them. In other words, in this dreamy realm the
fingers work in close formation as a daring company of corporeal,
intelligence-gathering scouts, gaining access to secret places, and
are clearly able to cover surprisingly long distances in no time
at all.

Most of us if we are scrupulously honest would acknowledge that the game of love shares many of the qualities of the
tournament. And at times we play for the highest emotional
stakes. Some of us are far better at it than others. Some of us
suffer from a succession of morale-crushing defeats, or even the
frustration of never being selected to play—but the metaphor is
ancient, and the trophy so attractive that few ever abandon the
competition entirely. And our quest to grasp that prize may at
times give rise to the suspicion that the prize and the adversary
are one and the same, the emotional equivalent of scaling a Co-
topaxi, Annapurna, or Everest—or ideally something or someone not quite as elevated.

The game of love is self-evidently also a form of performance. It requires the equivalent of practice and preparation,
an acute sense of timing—or if you lack that, then the ability to
navigate a wrong note, a missed cue, and to pick up the thread
once more as seamlessly as possible. You need confidence—if
not genuine confidence, then certainly the appearance of it—and
the ability to perform in front of an audience inevitably consisting
of at least a handful of people you know, and professional critics
whose opinions must be accepted for what they are. The game
of love is likewise sustained by the rhythms of time, unless it is
a form of unequal manipulation, or an expression of power, or
violence, or the product of extortion—in which case the teeth
and digits are fearfully prone to the demonizing imagery of fang

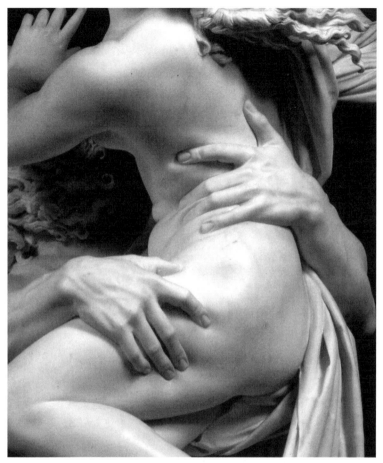

The fingers of Pluto pressing into the soft, warm flesh of Persephone makes this statue by Gianlorenzo Bernini one of the most breathtaking displays of technical virtuosity ever achieved in cold marble.

and claw, of unstoppable monsters such as Count Dracula—in other words, under relatively normal circumstances the erotic agency and exchange of human touch aspire to the condition not of loudly competing melodies, but of genuine polyphonic synthesis.

Young Richard Heber, the son of a well-to-do intellectually minded clergyman, grew up to become a passionate book collector, one of the leading bibliophiles of his generation, but at the game of love he was sadly inept. In the early 1820s, Heber's close friendship with the nineteen-year-old Charles Henry Hartshorne (1802–65) led to damaging rumors about a homosexual relationship between the two. Heber was twenty-nine years older than Hartshorne, and while still a schoolboy the younger man composed Latin verses for his charismatic friend. When in 1825 Heber suddenly resigned his seat in Parliament, it was claimed that he fled abroad just before a warrant was issued for his arrest on a charge of sodomitical practices. The Tory *John Bull* wrote: "Mr. Heber, the late Member for Oxford University, will not return to this country for some time—the backwardness of the season renders the Continent more congenial to some constitutions."

Heber's friend Sir Walter Scott feared the rumors were true, but no evidence has been found of any outstanding warrant.

NINE

The Finger of Combat

Blessed be the LORD my strength,
which teacheth my hands to war,
and my fingers to fight:
My goodness, and my fortress;
my high tower, and my deliverer;
my shield, and he in whom I trust;
who subdueth my people under me.

—Psalm 144:1–2

I hate the sight of men in their cups who shout, poke their fingers in
their mouths, stroke their beards, and pass on the wine to their neighbors with great cries of "Have some more! Drink up!"
—Sei Shōnagon (965–?1010s), from "Hateful Things," in
The Pillow Book, translated by Ivan I. Morris

"I asked them to show me modern art," she continued, "and I couldn't
see anything in it at all. The next time I began to understand." Suddenly
she jabbed a finger in my chest: *"See, see, see,"* she told me, *"learn, learn,
learn."* —Daniel Farson meets Lady Thatcher, summer 1993

I am proud of my driving. In the twenty-two years since I was
successfully taught to drive a car by that gruff but wise, indeed

redoubtable transplanted Englishman John Thomas, I have never had a ticket, nor to my knowledge been guilty of a misdemeanor while driving on either side of the road (right or left)—not on four continents, nor several islands offshore.

For those of us who are fastidious about staying in the correct lane the rewards are few. Nor does anybody thank us for prudently signaling well ahead of time, letting people enter from the left or right, or actually observing pedestrian crossings. Driving in as straight a line as possible (except when turning steadily, maybe even gracefully, as the lines on the road dictate); steering confidently but smoothly; operating the clutch and gears mindful of the requirements and well-being of the engine; neither holding up the traffic by driving too slowly on freeways, nor going much too fast; forgoing the convenience of driving while drunk, and also the spontaneity of the split-second mind-change—these practices seem at times almost quaint, while in many jurisdictions aggressive tailgating and indulging in no doubt enjoyable, foaming-spittle road rage are now sadly commonplace. People who scrupulously avoid both must nevertheless learn to accept them from other people, and for this almost superhuman degree of tolerance we may not expect to be given a medal.

I have found that when offered the gentle rebuke of a toot on the horn (for which purpose motor vehicles are equipped), persons who pass in the inside lane at recklessly high speed, brake suddenly, drift aimlessly at the brink of an intersection while attempting to decide what to do next, or otherwise behave erratically or dangerously—even when not being further distracted by cell phones—are much inclined to respond by proffering a gesture often as surprising as it is offensive. Regularly, they give us "the finger."

This ubiquitous gesture of defiance and contempt, indeed of anger, varies slightly from place to place. When I was growing up in Australia the index and middle fingers were raised together, sometimes even splayed, to form a gesture with identically the same meaning. That lingering Old World usage was presumably not unknown to Winston Churchill, who cannily chose to employ it also—often with cigar—as a convenient and potent if stubby approximation of the letter *V*, for Victory. Thanks to Douglas Ritchie, this practice soon found its way into the BBC European Radio service, which from 1941 until the end of the war used as its call sign a rhythmical approximation of the Morse code for *V*—three dots and a dash—ingeniously configured in the melody of the opening bars of Beethoven's Symphony no. 5 in C Minor (opus 67). Perhaps persuaded that its associations were too improper, Churchill gradually swiveled his famous *V* for Victory gesture around so that it more often came to be presented palm side out, and in that form during the mid-1960s it passed into the hands of a new generation, for whom the same gesture conveyed the counterculture messages of peace and love, while at the same time apparently still referencing *V*, but this time for Vietnam.

Since those halcyon days, the two-fingered iteration, which still persists in Britain, has in Australia been gradually supplanted by the longstanding American custom of presenting the rigidly extended, upwardly oriented distal phalanges of the middle finger only. The message is unambiguous, indeed unmistakable. It is what my friend Lynne Truss has described as the "eff off" injunction. And it is noteworthy that a gesture with such potent sexual implications should now be widely deployed so casually, it seems, by drivers of both sexes—and indeed by millions in less encumbered, infinitely variable contexts—when some call to combat in a public place seems justified, but nevertheless carefully contained.

People do not often give us the finger at dinner parties or in press conferences, or from the bench, pulpit, or throne (much as it may from time to time be sorely tempting for the occupant of each occasionally to do so). True, in these more formal contexts there may be subtler methods of conveying essentially the same message, but the finger is generally held in reserve. By contrast, many drivers seem so habituated to this particular language of silent abuse that they may not even bother to look in the direction in which it is cast. Indeed, this may well be one reason why it is so useful to so many. You can give someone the finger without taking your eyes off the road, and for small mercies I suppose we must be grateful.

There is, of course, a larger point, which comes to mind especially when the finger so rudely configured happens to be very youthful, arthritically gnarled, or decorated with the comely finial of a manicured and scrupulously lacquered fingernail, in which case the gesture may seem especially incongruous. Where do the very young pick these things up, and develop such blasé willingness so to address the blameless middle-aged? The very old should know better. And evidently prosperous mothers allow themselves the giddy pleasure of bidding us to go fuck ourselves from the driver's seat of a late-model Mercedes-Benz, with toddlers on board, safely strapped into their car seats.

To some extent these observations relate to the curious admixture of shared enterprise, solitariness, concentration, and hypnosis that characterizes such time as we spend immured in traffic, in many cases evidently a high proportion of the span of our daily lives. On the open road each of us is suspended for the time being in a convenient bubble, yet we also learn how to function automatically as a group. The vast majority of us know that our lives depend upon reading and responding without question to red lights, and as far as possible taking account of the trajectory of the other vehicles with which we rub shoulders, praying that they will not sideswipe, collide with, or explode on top of us. Fog, rain, and snow impose obvious limitations of which most drivers take account individually, but corporately also. Therefore, often it is some slight but irritating glitch in the communal aspect of our shared mission on the road, maybe even a maddening breakdown, that from the vantage point of our apparently secure and private cockpit emboldens us to give someone else the finger, safe in the knowledge that the recipient is unlikely to respond other than in kind. People who give us the finger mostly assume we will not use a crowbar to gain entry to their vehicle and exact some hideous sort of reprisal, at least not while they are traveling at speed. This assumption may not be justified. According to my copy of the State of Connecticut Department of Motor Vehicles *Driver's Manual*: "If you want to waive [*sic*] to another driver, please use all of your fingers, not just one. Obscene gestures have gotten people shot, stabbed, or beaten." Quite. And to make certain, I do not myself under any circumstances give other people the finger.

In any event, by resorting to the current syntax of gesture many people in our society (and not only drivers) seem more than content, often ebulliently determined, to express in this particular sexually explicit shorthand considerable amounts of hostility—despite the blunt but prudent advice of the Connecticut Department of Motor Vehicles. Occasionally, the obscene finger may be deployed in more nuanced ways, from the stage at crepuscular rock concerts, for example, or as a jocular demonstration to intimate acquaintances of what we wish more than anything we could with impunity express to telemarketers if they did not hover under the cowardly protection and anonymity of the telephone. In their wan quest, paparazzi are habituated to receiving "the finger" from starlets, hacks, and roués, though naturally this is useful grist for their particular mill. Indeed, apart from editors who from time to time acquire their photographs, paparazzi are among the very few people who actually receive "the finger" with genuine feelings of gladness.

Even more tribally, "the finger" seems not out of place at

sporting fixtures and heated political rallies, where the message
is counterbalanced if not by esprit de corps, then at least by the
latitude permitted by the general concepts of routine rough-
and-tumble, or of play, or else notional or apostrophized as distinct from hand-to-hand combat. There are other gestures that
even more explicitly refer to the act of coitus, such as the Italian
mano fica (a fistlike attitude with the thumb pushing suggestively
between the index and middle finger), or the even cruder index
finger of one hand poking through an *O* formed by opposing the thumb and index finger of the other—yet the immediate and underlying character of the canonical "finger" is always
more aggressively hostile, and phallic in origin and implication.
How did we arrive at this point? What does "the finger" in this
disturbingly sexualized, maybe even vaguely exciting context actually mean? For what form of restraint can we be grateful that
the vast majority of cross men who routinely present us with it
opt for the phallic finger, and not the male sex organ it represents? How do women feel about giving people the finger, if at
all differently?

The origins of "the finger" extend back at least as far as
Greco-Roman antiquity, where it is to be found in the comedies
of Aristophanes, and in numerous later Latin sources cheekily
popping up as the *digitus infamis* or *digitus impudicus*. Its explicit
sexual meaning was by then firmly established, and seems to
have taken as its cue the fact that the normal middle finger is
almost invariably the longest of the five, and therefore either
(a) the most satisfactory sexual stimulator; or (b) the proudest
as regards any implied declaration of the size of the gesturer's
own penis; or (c) in some way tied through association—and
by physical restraint, because it is very difficult to move one independently of the other—to the concept of the *digitus medicus*,
that is, the neighboring ring or "medical" finger, which was in a
different but evidently not unrelated context thought to represent the healing god Aesculapius.

In an ingenious and stinging invective against a man called Sextillus, the epigrammist Martial (2:28) urged his victim to use "the finger" against anyone who dared to call him a bugger, and, incidentally, ran through a catalog of other Roman sexual vices he claimed the poor man did not engage in, and by a process of elimination arrived at the two he clearly did:

> Go ahead and laugh at the man who calls you a queer,
> Sextillus, and give him the [middle] finger.
> But you aren't a bugger, Sextillus, no, nor a fucker,
> Nor does the hot cheek of Old Mama give you
>   pleasure.
> I confess you aren't one of these, Sextillus: Then what
>   are you?
> I don't know, but you know two things are left.

Those two things were evidently fellatio and cunnilingus. As regards "the finger," the ancient Roman usage was absolutely identical to ours.

Now, in ancient Greece life-sized humanoid sculptures known as herms were originally used to mark the boundaries of a sanctuary, and for other religious and commemorative functions. These were freestanding, downward-tapering square columns or plinths surmounted by a bearded human head (generally of Hermes, hence the name) but often also equipped with feet at the base and genitalia halfway up. So configured, the Roman equivalent of Hermes was Terminus, the god of boundaries and landmarks, hence the Latin variant of *herm*, the excitingly different *term*. Because terms were used more broadly as boundary markers on roads and in other places, the Romans generally omitted the genitalia. However, Greek herms still retained a specifically religious function, and were usually oriented outward so that the erect penis assumed a kind of apotropaic function, making of the male sex organ a forthright declaration of territorial integrity: Stay out or else. Similarly, in antiquity "the finger" appears to have been deployed against the evil eye as much as it was used as a gesture of defiance. In Rome (as we have seen) "the finger" also seems to have further doubled as a specific rebuttal of accusations or inferences of homosexuality, presumably in this context repudiating the act of sodomy, indeed turning it back upon the accuser.

It is not clear how the strictly upward orientation of the finger, which we now have to tolerate, came to be the dominant mode, because certainly in ancient Rome more often than not it seems to have been poked *out*, not *up*. By combining in this sensible manner the *infamis/impudicus* message and the more straightforward function of pointing, you could presumably be far clearer about the identity of the person to whom you were determined to deliver it. Strangely, there seems to be absolutely no survival anywhere in our time of this outward-pointing form of obscene gesture; anthropologists have scrupulously recorded many forms of pointing all over the world, but as far as I can see, although they are occasionally construed as impolite, even rude, they are nowhere any longer understood to be obscene.

Nor was this Roman gesture, though explicitly sexual, readily associated with any related or indeed unrelated expressions of pure anger. According to the nineteenth-century German classicist Carl Sittl, angry Romans were far more likely to *bite* their fingers or nails as a public demonstration of wrath than to deploy the obscene finger, which, contrasting with the muddled usage of our era, seems to have been held strictly in reserve for exclusively obscene and/or semimagical purposes, and not as some conduit for wholly unerotic forms of aggression. One of the most frequently cited and misunderstood instances of the use of "the finger" in antiquity is that of Emperor Caligula. The story is told by Suetonius, toward the end of his brief but influential post hoc life of the corrupt emperor, when putting in context the assassination conspiracy:

The conspirators having resolved to fall upon the emperor as he returned at noon from the Palatine games, Cassius Chaerea, tribune of the Praetorian guards, claimed the part of making the onset. This Chaerea was now an elderly man, and had been often reproached by Caius [Caligula] for effeminacy. When he [Chaerea] came for the watchword, Caligula would give "Priapus," or "Venus"; and if on any occasion he [Chaerea] returned thanks, [Caligula] would offer him his hand to kiss, making with his fingers an obscene gesture.

A better English translation of the key phrase in Suetonius' smooth Latin is "he would hold out his hand to kiss, *forming and moving it in an obscene fashion*," which more accurately identifies Caligula's gesture as an unequivocally degrading insult and provocation, but essentially dismissive, contemptuous, and certainly not one of anger, or else, knowing what others thought about the bestial Caligula, Chaerea would certainly not have survived. Only a foolhardy or insane Roman emperor would play such a dangerous game with the commanding officer of his elite bodyguard, and, of course, the conspiracy—much fortified by favorable omens—was in due course successfully carried out. According to Suetonius, the insult to Chaerea was returned with interest when with their swords the Praetorian guards struck Caligula through the private parts. The literary point was that the emperor's (at best) jocular, very public, and carefully administered gesture of contempt—a breathtaking instance, moreover, of the pot calling the kettle black—was for him a hubristic point of no return.

Most cultures seem to have developed something like "the finger," and variants are numerous. In Sri Lanka, for example, it is the index and not the middle finger that is raised, and for some reason in Persia and Afghanistan it is the extended thumb. In the

Arab world, where any such gesture is far more unacceptable than in the West, it exists also, but the outer phalanges of the middle finger are apparently bent or folded in toward the palm rather than upraised, a curious nod toward modesty, though not enough of one to prevent the gesture from being deployed at all.

And there exists in many places a longstanding amplification of "the finger" into the entire forearm defiantly held aloft, fist clenched, at times emphatically supported by the other hand brought chopping down into the crook of the elbow. The meaning of this gesture is identically the same as that of "the finger," and it has a long history also. It crops up in Dutch painting of the seventeenth century, where thankfully it seems to be entirely jocular, no less frankly sexual, but essentially playful in complexion. I suppose it is not hard to see why the quantum leap from finger to whole forearm would strike some men as not merely logical but an especially satisfactory enlargement of the original gesture, and of course it has the advantage of being more clearly visible from much farther away. In this respect it may also reflect a measure of innate cowardice, since the far greater distance between gesturer and recipient necessarily yields a convenient envelope of time and space in which to make a hasty departure should the other man's reaction make this necessary. (I am not aware of any women who have habitually employed this form of gesture outside the domestic environment.) For anyone balancing on the knife's edge of honor and morality in seventeenth-century Europe we should assume that any such insult was not likely to go unnoticed.

What is so interesting about these observations about "the finger" and obscenity is that they are now ceaselessly discussed in chat rooms, forums, blogs, and other places on the Internet, usually harvesting and regurgitating the same inaccurate or garbled information lately accumulated on the pertinent Wikipedia page, where suburban legends find similarly rich nourishment.

Again and again the claim is made, for instance, that "the finger" acquired its current meaning as a gesture of defiance among long-bowmen during the Hundred Years' War, who rightly or wrongly, so the story goes, feared that the French, anticipating victory, meant to lop off the middle or bow finger of all captured English archers so as to make it impossible for them ever again to shoot arrows. In this context, "the finger" is dressed up as an archer's defiant battlefield gesture toward a potentially barbaric enemy, and a warning that his bow finger was intact and ready for action. It is hard to fathom how these myths originate, then spread and achieve such widespread currency, but the fact that a military and not an obscene derivation is now so widely sought suggests that the *digitus impudicus* arouses much anxiety in our time; if its origins may be construed as asexual, so much the better.

Of course, this current preoccupation with the middle fingers of longbowmen serves as a sobering reminder that before our era all combat was hand-to-hand, and the same skills of manual dexterity that gave us musical performance, and all literature, mathematics, agriculture, and works of art, were actually deployed for the far less beautiful purpose of clobbering our enemies. The rich but slightly tedious literature relating to "the arts of personal combat" insists that like a cold vulture wheeling over the head of man, violence has been with us from the very beginning. What has changed, of course, is that whereas the soldiers at Troy, Thermopylae, the Milvian Bridge, indeed at Agincourt, were invited to bring those skills into direct and theoretically fair competition with opponents more or less equally equipped—if not with the same measure of skill or armor, then certainly with the same general requirements of warfare—by a ghastly process of drift humanity has broadened the scope of violence almost infinitely so that we now live in global dread of chemical and biological weapons, to say nothing of vast explosions, the use of which entirely disregards the idea of the killing of innocent bystanders or any other sort of ruinous collateral damage. It is of no comfort at all to reflect that these evils generally require the finger of a hopefully cogent individual to depress the relevant button or wire the pertinent fuses.

We were evidently a species well accustomed in times of more "primitive" warfare to heinous eye-gouging; lethal stone-throwing; club, mace, dagger, sword, and pike-wielding; and arrow-shooting—sometimes with extraordinary skill, incidentally also dragging with us into vicious battles that gentle, intelligent, grass-eating creature the horse. More recently, with the coming of gunpowder, we developed the sharp hand-to-eye coordination that makes the combination of index finger and the trigger of a loaded musket, rifle, or revolver so lethal. In other words, we bludgeoned, strangled, garroted, mutilated, tortured, dueled, stabbed, knuckle-dusted, shot, and fired our way to victory or defeat, but there was, at least in theory, a sharp division between the occasions upon which those activities were legitimately placed at our disposal (and held in check by military commanders), and when the use of them against innocent noncombatants in peacetime was regarded as a terrible evil. True, there has always been a question mark hanging over the disposition of the line that separates the martial from the criminal—never more so than during the Counter-Reformation in Europe, or the conquest of the New World—but before the advent of explosives we were thankfully constrained by the simple fact that the amount of damage we could do to other people was restricted by the number of individual soldiers our princes and generals had at their disposal. So the gradual industrialization of warfare has brought us to the point at which the detonating finger of a single person may obliterate entire cities, and the trigger fingers of comparatively few can and have dispatched millions, whole populations. In the circumstances, it is little short of amazing that we should have turned archery and shooting into Olympic sports, and entirely baffling that we are now so willing to place lethal firearms at the disposal of nearly anyone who satisfies those few lax regulations that are, it seems, held permanently in check by the relevant portion of the Second Amendment of the United States Constitution. The truly astonishing thing is not so much that there are so many gun-related deaths in America—29,569 in 2004 alone, of which almost 12,000 were homicides, more than 16,750 suicides, and approximately 650 accidental deaths, which adds up to about 80 gun-related deaths on every day of that year—but rather that there are not many, many more. How much more remarkable, then, that mindful of the awesome breadth of human weakness, our consistent propensity toward violence and proneness to the most desperate passions, we should apparently regard the exchange of *any* threat or insult, even one as apparently benign or trivial as "the finger," as an unremarkable aspect of daily life, to be disregarded or responded to as the case may be.

Nor am I sure if we may derive any encouragement or reassurance at all from the fact that "the finger" is mostly reined in by quotation marks—quotation marks, moreover, with which these days many people seem more and more willing to decorate their speech, in other words, by deploying that slightly irritating twin gesture consisting of the uplifted wiggling index and middle fingers of both hands (as if to say "This is not exactly the right word or phrase I seek, so please be aware that a better one ought to go between these inverted commas, but I cannot for the time being think of what it is"). Although we have seen how eloquent the formal languages of gesture can be, and how accurate, they are by their nature apostrophized, shorthand gestures, especially very widespread, hold-all gestures such as "the finger," which combines symbolic elements of defiance and obscenity (above all the idea of sexual penetration)—these inevitably gain entry to the mind of the person on the receiving end quite as effectively as we scrupulously avoid penetrating the same person's own body.

Given the potency of that particular combination of deep sensitivities, there can be no guarantees that when we give someone "the finger" he will not respond as at length Chaerea did to Caligula. True, we live in a society that has over the past fifty years shown an admirable capacity to expand in tolerance. Maybe depending upon where you live, these days you are probably less likely to be held up to ridicule or even attacked on the grounds of race or sexual orientation or religious affiliation than was once the case, but it is also true that fear and suspicion of the foreign, the hatefully and irreconcilably different, or the plain revolting run very, very deep. There are absolutely no guarantees that unlike earlier generations we are immune to them. The difference, however, is that where they dwell now they tend to dwell in secret, successfully silenced by higher standards of public behavior (even legislation). Nevertheless, they exist. They are nourished by paranoia, insecurity, and self-loathing. They occupy discreet emotional crannies of unnatural hate, whence in the fullness of time poisonous creepers, leathery parasitic vines, the tendrils of stinking Rhinanthus duly sprout, their twisting suckers nourished by years of loneliness, watered with resentment from salten creek beds, richly fertilized by private anger. If giving someone "the finger" is a tiny valve on that emotional pressure cooker, I suppose it is not just to be tolerated, but maybe even encouraged. Yet something tells the historian in me that, where it flourishes, and as often as it is resorted to, that same hostile finger is also depressing a small, metaphorical, but nevertheless insistent alarm bell.

From my study window I derive much pleasure from watching Connecticut motorists attempting to parallel park. It is not a difficult maneuver, as John Thomas once pointed out to me.

Align yourself appropriately with the car in front of the vacant spot, change gear into reverse, turn the wheel, and, using your external driver's-side rearview mirror to calculate the right angle, attain the orientation needed to insert your hindquarters snugly into the vacant spot. Adjust your trajectory (crucial), and continue to move steadily backward *in a straight line*, then, turning the wheel in the other direction, complete the exercise so that you bring yourself into exactly parallel alignment with the curb, prudently leaving enough space for the people in front and behind you to extract themselves in due course. In so many respects parallel parking is like life; you ought to be able to achieve what is necessary in one go.

Unfortunately, in Connecticut—I am not familiar with the practices of other states—the only parking requirement in the current driving test is for the candidate to enter a parking lot, make a simple ninety-degree turn, and drift nose-first into a wide, empty space, a straightforward maneuver of which surely few are incapable, even though many vehicles thus deposited outside supermarkets and railroad stations often seem not parked so much as abandoned.

So from where I sit I see a daily, hourly procession of drivers heave their back wheel onto the curb, bang into the car behind them, or make do with Lewis and Clark–level distances separating their vehicles from the sidewalk. Even if finally successful, many motorists come up with playfully novel working definitions of the word *parallel*.

There is nothing as unnerving, when trying to achieve something difficult, as suddenly becoming aware that you are being watched, and with considerable amusement. So it is just now with the portly woman in the large silver Buick who for several minutes has been worrying that the ample margin of at least six long feet separating the relevant portion of her bumper from the mountainous Hummer in front is plainly insufficient. Hers is a simple miscalculation buoyed by excessive caution, but comical nonetheless. Some people make several zigzagging attempts to parallel park, persisting with creditable pluck and determination, apparently approaching this task in the spirit of experimentation, even adventure and free enterprise. Others simply give up.

She has just now noticed that from the safety and comfort of my snug vantage point I am transfixed by her deepening dilemma, chuckling quietly to myself. In a sense I am actually with her, sending forth encouraging vibrations, hoping she will manage to get there in the end. However, my portly motorist with the Alice band does not see me in this kindly light. She has much to do, little time, and even less patience. Swinging forthrightly into the road, she sinks her foot onto the accelerator and roars off, but not before giving me "the finger."

O tempora, o mores.

TEN

The Strange Status of the Thumb

By the pricking of my thumbs,
Something wicked this way comes.
Open, locks, whoever knocks!
> —William Shakespeare, *Macbeth*,
> c. 1603–06, act IV, sc. i

O bounce! O flea! How sharp you bite!
I think far more of you to-night
Than of aught else beneath the moon,
Ay, or beyond it. But how soon
I shall forget!—ev'n should I fail
To catch you on my fierce thumb-nail.
> —William Allingham, from "Blackberries," 1890

We spend more grey matter in the brain manipulating the thumb than in the total control of the chest and the abdomen.
> —Jacob Bronowski, *The Ascent of Man*, 1973

This book began with a simple question: Is the thumb a finger? Hopefully that question was answered unequivocally at the very outset with a resounding yes. But more than this, it is the dependable thumb and its opposability with each of the other four fingers—a capacity for motion that is unique to the human hand—that have elevated mankind to our current position at the top of the evolutionary tree.

All of us know, or think we know, if only from constantly accumulating experience, exactly what we can and cannot do with our hands and our fingers—even the sedentary, whose thumbs are nowadays especially busy "texting," or, in the case of those too lazy even to bother with vowels, sending "txts." However, anatomists have provided us with a convenient language with which to isolate with great precision each type of motion of which our hands are capable. The relevant terms are rational, Latin-dependent, and at times tedious, but by guiding us toward and pinning down specifics, they serve the useful purpose of shedding shafts of light on the whole mechanism in all its magnificence.

Abduction, as the more common, criminal usage of the word suggests, is the movement of a part of the body *away* from an imaginary straight line that passes, if we are talking about limbs, from the top of your head, down through the middle of your body to a spot on the ground between your feet, like a plumb line. The *adduction* of a limb is the opposite, a movement back toward that line. As applied to the hand, only our fingers, the phalanges, and the proximal edge of the wrist are capable of those movements, which relate instead to a different imaginary straight line that runs down through the middle of your forearm and wrist, and shoots out the tip of your middle finger—if, and only if, you are sitting at a table that is approximately the height of your elbow and your hand is placed flat on it, the palm facing downward, relaxed or at rest. For the time being, let us adopt this calming position, and proceed.

In simple terms, if you go ahead and now spread or splay your fingers as far as you can and then return them to the position of rest, we have essentially performed the actions of abduction (movement away), then adduction (movement back again), with the possible exception of the middle finger, which—I am guessing—probably stayed in about the same spot. Now, if you tinker a little you will notice that you ought to be able to move each digit from side to side individually. Without this fundamental skill we would lack the entire corpus of Western keyboard music, and much else besides.

Extension and flexion are similarly paired types of movement, which likewise relate to the change in angle between two bones that meet at a joint. But this time these movements "hinge" on imaginary lines that run more or less at right angles to the one I mentioned earlier. Technically, when you flex your biceps you are not performing an elaborate mating dance in a Chelsea gymnasium but instead *decreasing* the angle formed by the junction of bones at your elbow. Now, to go back to your hand, which I trust is still resting on the table, let us perform a little experiment by making a claw. This is unattractive, but I am afraid necessary. What you have done is to flex certain muscles so as to decrease the angle between each of the interphalangeal joints. Flexion has occurred.

Now reverse that motion, and try to carry it as far as you can in the opposite direction, so that as well as being straightened out, your fingers (with luck) are now lifted off the table, and only the fleshy mounds at the base of your fingers will be touching the tasteful tablecloth, stylish white oak, or whatever your table is made of. Houston, we have extension. Now relax, and put your fingers back in the "rest" position. Notice, incidentally, that in this "make-a-claw-then-not-merely-unravel-it-but-keep-going-and-stretch-your-fingers-back-as-far-as-you-possibly-can-without-forcing-them-then-comma-finally-comma-relax" experiment, in all probability you are combining many flexion, extension, abduction, and adduction movements in suave combination without even realizing it. If you concentrate carefully, you ought to be able to repeat the exercise and exclude the motions of abduction and adduction, in which case the two positions you attain will remind you, first, of scooping a hole in the sand on a beach and, second, of a sort of military salute.

Opposition is a unique action of the human hand that allows you to bring the tip of your thumb into many different types of contact with all of the remaining fingers and fingertips, either singly or in combination. The most vital parts of this action in fact occur at the joints between the wrist, or carpal, bones and the metacarpals, of which the shortest and most important supports the thumb.

If you are right-handed and you now go ahead and thread a needle, in all likelihood you have opposed the thumb and index finger of your left hand so that the needle is held firmly between the tips. I gather that there are some in the Garment District who might opt for the more elegant opposition of thumb and middle finger for securing the needle, but that is neither here nor there. The thumb and index finger of your right hand, meanwhile, are similarly opposed so as to manipulate the thread, chartreuse cotton, perhaps. Now, and we are starting to see more shafts of manual sunshine, you will observe if you do it again in slow motion that the needle-threading exercise involves not merely the opposition of thumb and index finger but, particularly in the case of your right hand, certain precise combined actions of finger flexion, extension, abduction (see what the other fingers are doing?), and, afterward, graceful adduction arising from pleasure in a job well done.

Finally, none of these capacities for motion would extend much further than basic robotics or, to shift for a moment to a theatrical metaphor, equip your hand with more than the versatility required of, say, the more inert roles in Noh theater or Samuel Beckett, unless our arm and wrist were endowed with the capacities of pronation and supination, which in turn rely on the ability of the radius and ulna, the bones of the forearm, to cross, change position in relation to each other, and bring about motions in the wrist of swiveling and rotation. All the foregoing motions of the distal parts of the hand thus acquire from this fundamental, "root-and-branch" point of contact between the wrist and the arm that versatility, strength, delicacy, accuracy, and sheer range of motion we expect, demand of, and applaud in a great prima ballerina.

So, in a nutcracker, reverting to the tabletop, if your left hand is resting facedown, try to flip it over to the palm-upward position. You will find that you can successfully do this unaided only by rotating your wrist in one direction. That motion is called supination, and is the consequence of uncrossing the radius and ulna. Believe it or not, the anatomists tell us that after you have done this, and you are gazing at your palm, your hand is said to be supine, that is, prone, or, for reasons that should not detain us, adopting the "anatomical" position. Now flip it back again and, congratulations, you have performed the motion called pronation: your ulna and radius are now deftly crossed.

In every case, limitations are imposed upon the motions set in train by muscles and tendons both by the structure of the bones themselves (that is, your wrist will not rotate, or pronate, any further because if it did the bones in your arm and/or wrist would either break, or the joints dislocate) and by the ligaments (that is, your index finger will not bend back or extend any further because if it did, either the phalanges would break or certain ligaments would tear), and in all instances the pertinent nerve endings would, unless somehow compromised (but let us not dally), alert you to this fact with considerable urgency. In an instant your muscle, joint, and other receptors will have sent urgent messages up the long neurological pathway to the brain, to which an immediate response is required: Ouch. These observations have not been lost on those miserable persons who continue to practice the ancient arts of torture, and await higher judgment.

Most if not all infants suck their thumbs, and it was a curious byproduct of the rapid development of pediatric medicine in the nineteenth century that this innate tendency soon came to be regarded with dark foreboding as pathological. If babies were permitted to suck their thumbs, and suck to their heart's content, all kinds of dire consequences could be expected. Pediatricians warned of ghastly dental malformation, problems with the soft palate, arrested development of speech, and above all, irregular patterns of sexual behavior later on. Leaving aside the obvious point that its natural position, convenient shortness, and winsome ease of access to the mouth make the thumb an ideal source of comfort for a baby, it seems unlikely that if Victorian doctors had taken the trouble to consult nursemaids, nannies, or, incidentally, mothers, they would have made quite as much as they did of the dangers of thumb-sucking. Nor would they have been so willing to build on this wildly improbable foundation such a haunted house of cards as in due course rose up around the concept of masturbation in adults. Nevertheless, thumb-sucking burrowed its reliable way into many textbooks of pediatric medicine in the last quarter of the nineteenth century, and persisted well into the twentieth. The issue was still controversial in the 1950s when a vigorous correspondence in *The Times* arose from remarks reported from a meeting of child psychologists in Oxford:

> They were somewhat startled at the end of the morning to hear that, as nearly 50 per cent of normal [seven-year-old] children indulge in thumb-sucking, there is not much to worry about... Amplifying his statement, [Dr. R. G. McInnes] said that thumb-sucking was a pleasant and harmless way of passing the time until the next meal came round, and in any case it deserved the same consideration as that achieved by smokers at a later age. A well sucked thumb was much less toxic than a pipe which had seen some service.

This sanguine assessment drew an angry retort from a dentist in Dorking, Surrey:

Before making carefree remarks about thumb-sucking, Dr. McInnes ... might have considered the damage and deformity caused to the maxilla by this habit, resulting in much tedious work for the orthodontist, and patient wearing of appliances by young children. All this can be avoided by the breaking of this harmful habit.

In due course the doughty Scottish matron of Davington School at Usk in Monmouthshire responded with a dose of good sense. The particular emphasis of the final sentence improves greatly if you imagine it spoken with a strong accent:

Observation teaches me that 50 per cent. of children may suck their thumbs, but that in all probability it has no effect on their teeth. Some children who are habitual thumb-suckers cause no deformation; others who virtually never do so have protruding second teeth. I know intimately two children of the same family, both of whom require treatment by the orthodontist for similar deformations. One was of the 50 per cent. of thumb-suckers; in the other the habit was conspicuously lacking.

These days we may feel the effortless superiority of later generations who know better, but this focus on thumb-sucking, this unreasonable fear of it, was a striking feature of the formal study of pediatrics until remarkably recently, and dissipated almost as suddenly as it first appeared in Harley Street. True, one may now be surprised to observe adolescents or even adults sucking their thumbs, but in the society we have created for ourselves there now seem so many more desperate things than that for doctors to be concerned about.

Just as for most of us now living in civilized communities our consultation with an appropriately qualified medical practitioner begins, or certainly ought to, with a handshake, not too firm, not too limp, among many experienced doctors that interaction constitutes far more than a polite greeting. It is an opportunity for them to make the first of what are often extremely telling diagnostic observations. A tremor in the hand, or worse, delirium tremens (known as DTs, for short), will allow the patient not merely to say "Hello," but also to announce himself as an alcoholic, a seasoned abuser of benzodiazepines or barbiturates (and in need of more, *now*), or a chronic tobacco smoker, the sides of his index and middle fingers prettily coated with amber, yellow, and brown nicotine stains. Meanwhile, a horrid thing called a spider nevus was first observed disfiguring the skin of an aggressively tippling nineteenth-century English publican, and also white nail beds; either of these may indicate low albumen, malnutrition, anemia, or liver failure, either pending, in process, or very nearly attained.

Abnormal contractions or paralyses; genetic glitches such as polydactyly (extras), syndactyly (that is, digits that failed to separate in utero), or some rare forms of "webbing"; missing fingers (Frostbite? Is this one of those people, a bit of a lad, who is too tough, reckless, or stoical to take proper care of himself?); clubbing—not the nocturnal variety, but that of the fingernails—to say nothing of the disorder known as Dupuytren's contracture, which among other disorders can provide early indications of alcohol abuse or incipient heart disease; encephalopathic "flapping"; tiny subungual splinters (that is, under the nails); fingernails anxiously bitten to the quick, or beyond; bleeding; wasting; or bruising; any one of these may alert the doctor to dirty work at the pathological or even psychological crossroads, or something as basic as domestic violence.

All of these may be observed in an instant on our hands and fingers by those doctors who can now bear to take their eyes off the flickering blue light of the computer screen, and I doubt if any medical practitioner worth his salt would not wish to compare the gloomy data extracted from blood samples with what he sees sitting nervously in the chair on the other side of his desk. It is those wise owls who use their eyes and, incidentally, exploit the sensitivity of their fingertips, who can and will continue to discover much in their patients' handshake.

Some basic methods of the physical examination of patients by Western doctors have not changed much in recent centuries, and, of course, feeling for lumps, bumps, hardness, or roughness, with varying degrees of precision, has been a standard skill exercised by doctors since antiquity. Indeed, recent work on methods of divination in ancient Greece shows how closely the methods of the doctor resembled those of the seer, the main difference being that as well as closely observing the flight of birds (the *auspices*), seers examined dead livers while doctors prodded about for healthy human ones; both exploited as far as possible the sense of touch, and exercised the considerable skills of discrimination they had at their fingertips.

A more recent method of physical examination, and comforting because of the satisfactory resonance of the sound it produces from a healthy chest, is percussion: the tap-tap-tapping of the doctor's index and middle fingers of one hand against the dorsal side of the other, placed flat on the patient's back, chest, or abdomen. This diagnostic procedure was discovered and published in the mid–eighteenth century by Leopold Auenbrugger, the son of a Viennese wine merchant, who, as a child, watched his father use a similar method to gauge the declining level of wine in his barrels. Auenbrugger was a doctor in the Spanish Hospital in Vienna, and over seven years made careful observations of the sounds produced when percussing the chests of his patients. Because he was also in charge of carrying out postmortem examinations when at length they died, evidently in quite large numbers, Auenbrugger was able to reach firm conclusions about what a healthy chest cavity ought to sound like, and that,

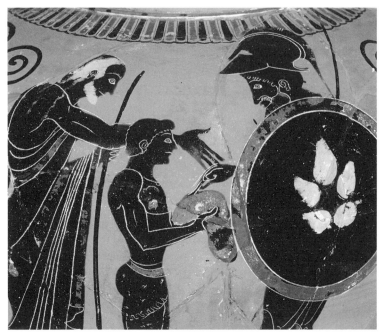

In ancient Greece, the methods of diagnosis employed by the doctor and divination by the seer were strikingly similar. Here an Attic youth presents the liver of a sacrificial victim to a bearded hoplite for careful examination.

for example, abnormal growths, masses, or tumors in the lung produced a dull sound, as against the distinctly deeper resonance produced by healthy lungs. Auenbrugger's discovery of percussion, which was originally published in 1761, and which led very indirectly to the invention of the stethoscope, took a long time to become widely known. Although the book appears to have been reviewed anonymously in London by Oliver Goldsmith, it was not until 1806, when Napoleon's physician, Jean-Nicolas Corvisart, adopted the method in his clinical practice in Paris that Auenbrugger's major contribution to the art of modern medicine was widely recognized.

In the fraught realm of human relationships it is important to remember that the handshake is one of our most precious assets, and (apart from the curious gesture now known as "high fives"—but the name implies that the thumb at least joins in) a handshake cannot be exchanged without the enclosing clasp of the thumb. Yet even to come into physical contact with a hand in fully working order was until remarkably recently a physical encounter apt to be subjected to harsh moral judgment, and one suspects at times it still is. In 1873, for example, the Harvard Unitarian Cyrus Augustus Bartol took a firm line on hands to be avoided:

> There is a hand that has no heart in it, there is a claw or paw, a flipper or fin, a bit of wet cloth to take hold of, a piece of unbaked dough on the cook's trencher, a cold clammy thing we recoil from, or greedy clutch with the heat of sin, which we drop like a burning coal. What a scale from the talon to the horn of plenty is this human palm leaf! Sometimes it is like a knife-shaped, thin-bladed tool we dare not grasp, or like a poisonous thing we shake off, or unclean member, which, white as it may look, we feel polluted by.

While these days we may regard nineteenth-century severities spilling from a Boston pulpit as quaint or frankly absurd, and incidentally note their racist hint, I suspect if we are scrupulously honest one or two of these images may for quite a lot of us still ring a faint but disturbingly clear bell, and cause a corresponding degree of discomfiture.

Even more surprising is the practice, reported in 1863 by the London *Saturday Review*, of presenting only two fingers as an acceptable substitute for a handshake consisting of all five:

> There are people in England to be met with every day who have a horrid habit of giving two fingers only when they pretend to shake hands. They use this means to express the feeling of their own importance, and also to convey to the person on whom they confer this doubtful honour a proper sense of the distance that separates them. Fine ladies in the country not unfrequently hold out this signal of their consequence to creatures like curates, attorneys, younger sons, and led captains; and from the affable smile with which they accompany the gesture it is evident that they seriously believe those kind of people must be pleased and proud to have this mark of condescension shown them...Many of those, however, who have the two fingers pushed into their hand are stung with the implication of inferiority, and do not like this trait in the manners of their superiors. Sometimes they even threaten to give what they get, and to offer two fingers in return.

Fortunately, this frightful practice seems to have withered on the vine, but it is certainly true that an especially limp or else a ferociously overbearing handshake can make a strong impact upon what subsequently transpires between new acquaintances.

Yet I wonder how often those of us fortunate enough to have at our disposal a full set of fingers and above all a fully opposable thumb ever imagine functioning without it?

As we have seen, the Romans were inclined to associate the thumb, *pollex*, with sexual potency, but more generally with physical strength, and whether or not ancient speculation about the Latin etymology was correct (maybe from *polleo, -ere*, to be strong or powerful), they certainly had the right general idea. The thumb is powerful indeed, as a sensory outrider to the hand, as a durable support, as an indispensable component of grip, and as the digit that makes all the rest such effective tools. And perhaps the right note on which to close is to consider its larger significance, its cheerful posture as an upraised sign of approbation, much reinforced with a smile.

Many people believe that the gesture of "thumbs down" owes its existence to the practice of using it to determine the grisly fate of the victim of an ancient Roman gladiatorial contest. Certainly a gesture of the thumb was used by the crowd as a collective expression of opinion, but there is no better example than this of the supreme ambiguity of the ancient sources. Juvenal referred to the gladiator who wins applause "by slaying whoever the mob urges them to slay with *a turn of the thumb*" but maddeningly leaves unanswered the question as to precisely which direction the condemnatory thumb pointed. Up or down? In his stupendously vulgar set piece *Pollice Verso*, the French Orientalist painter Jean-Léon Gérôme opted firmly for *down*, and similarly potboiling efforts to reconstruct daily life in ancient Rome struggled to interpret this Latin phrase, which, strictly speaking, translates simply as "turn" but stops short of stipulating any particular direction. In a radically different context, Quintilian carefully described a gesture of threat in the following terms: "There is also a gesture, which consists in inclining the head to the right shoulder, stretching out the arm from the ear and extending the

hand *with the hostile thumb.* This is a special favorite with those
who boast that they speak 'with uplifted hand.'" This does not
help us at all, because while uplifted, the hand delivering that
"hostile thumb" obviously has the option of pointing it in any
direction through at least 270 degrees, up, down, or sideways. An
explicitly stated connection between this "hostile thumb" and
what went on in the Colosseum does not come until the sixth
century C.E., when it crops up in a collection of stray poems:
"Even in the fierce arena the conquered gladiator has hope, although the crowd threatens *with its hostile thumb.*"

The nearest thing we have to an explicit Roman statement
of thumb "direction" comes in Pliny, who mentions that "there is
even a proverb that bids us *turn down our thumbs to show approval.*"
It seems to have been on this basis that Charlton T. Lewis and
Charles Short, the compilers of the decidedly messy nineteenth-
century *Latin to English Lexikon* (1879), came firmly down on
the side of "thumbs up" for condemnation, and "thumbs down"
for reprieve. The ancient Romans certainly used gestures of this
general type in the Colosseum, but the real and overriding question is what approval actually meant in that ghastly arena. In
other words, "thumbs down" might well signify the wishes of
the crowd in respect to the fate of the defeated gladiator, and as
regards some perceived or actual blood-lust entertainment value,
either (a) "we approve" and "curtains," or (b) "we do *not* approve" and "curtains," or, for that matter, (c) "we approve" or
(d) "we do *not* approve" and "spare the poor bastard."

The best we can say is that it must have been one of these
four, or else the right combination was indicated instead by the
gesture of "thumbs up." We shall almost certainly never know.
The fact that this question now stirs so much interest among
classical scholars and people more generally interested in the
customs, saws, and sayings of ancient Rome reveals a measure
of determination to double-check and shore up the upraised

thumb of current usage, the thumb that says "Ready to go," the thumb that says "Great," or "I couldn't be in better health or frame of mind, thank you very much." In the unlikely event that this book should survive the next two thousand years, it may yet serve a useful purpose by disclosing to whatever civilization is then prospering that in our era we deliberately chose not to use a gesture of the thumb to condemn wounded gladiators to a hideous death, but sought instead occasionally to deploy it as a friendly message of optimism, hope, or the cheerful reassurance of a kept promise, and a big task brought finally to completion.

Notes

Abbreviations

A   Richard Allsopp, ed., *Dictionary of Caribbean English Usage*. Oxford: Oxford University Press, 1996.

AND   W. S. Ramson, ed., *The Australian National Dictionary*. Melbourne: Oxford University Press, 1988.

B   Ivor H. Evans, ed., *Brewer's Dictionary of Phrase and Fable*. 2nd (revised) edition. London: Cassell, 1981.

B2   David Pickering et al., comps., *Brewer's Dictionary of 20th-Century Phrase and Fable*. London: Cassell, 1992.

B3   Adrian Room, comp., *Brewer's Dictionary of Modern Phrase and Fable*, London: Cassell, 2000.

B&B   Lester V. Berry and Melvin van den Bark, *The American Thesaurus of Slang, with Supplement: A Complete Reference Book of Colloquial Speech*. New York: Thomas Y. Cromwell Company, 1942.

Bozz   Mary Marshall, *Bozzimacoo: Origins & Meanings of Oaths & Swear Words*. Walton-on-Thames and London: M. & J. Hobbs, in association with Michael Joseph, 1975.

DA   "Ducange Anglicus" (pseud.), *The vulgar tongue: a glossary of slang, cant, and flash words and phrases, used in London from 1839 to 1859*. 2nd edition. London: B. Quaritch, 1859.

F&H   John Stephen Farmer and W. E. Henley, *Slang and its analogues, past and present. A dictionary, historical and comparative, of the heterodox speech of all classes of society for more than three hundred years* (1890–1904). 7 vols. New York: Kraus Reprint Corp., 1965.

Fowler   John Burchfield, *Fowler's Modern English Usage*. Revised 3rd edition. Oxford: Oxford University Press, 1998.

HM   Henry Mayhew, *London Labour and the London Poor: The Condition and Earnings of Those That Will Work, Cannot Work, and Will Not Work*. 3 vols. London: Charles Griffin and Co., 1951.

I&M   George Ingram (pseud.) and De Witt Mackenzie, *Hell's Kitchen. The story of London's underworld as related by the notorious ex-burglar George Ingram.* London: Herbert Jenkins, 1930.

JCH   J[ohn]. C[amden]. Hotten, *Dictionary of Modern Slang, Cant, and Vulgar Words, used at the present day in the streets of London; the universities of Oxford and Cambridge; the houses of Parliament; the dens of St. Giles; and the palaces of St. James.* London: J. C. Hotten, 1859.

JRW   J[ames]. Redding Ware, *Passing English of the Victorian era, a dictionary of heterodox English, slang, and phrase.* London: G. Routledge & Sons, 1909.

JW   Joseph Wright, *English Dialect Dictionary: Being the complete vocabulary of all dialect words still in use, or known to have been in use during the last two hundred years.* London: Henry Frowde, 1905.

NYT   *The New York Times*

ODNB Colin Matthew and Brian Harrison, eds., *Oxford Dictionary of National Biography.* Oxford University Press, 2004.

OED   J. A. Simpson and E. S. C. Weiner, eds., *The Oxford English Dictionary.* 2nd edition. Oxford: Oxford University Press (Clarendon Press), 1989.

Partridge   Eric Partridge, *A Dictionary of Slang and Unconventional English from the Fifteenth Century to the Present Day.* 5th edition. New York: Macmillan, 1961.

Partridge 2   Eric Partridge, *A Dictionary of the Underworld, British and American, Being the Vocabularies of Crooks, Criminals, Racketeers, Beggars and Tramps, Convicts, the Commercial Underworld, the Drug Traffic, the White Slave Traffic, Spivs.* 3rd edition. London: Routledge & Kegan Paul.

POB   *The Proceedings of the Old Bailey, London 1674 to 1834.* Sheffield, U.K., and Ann Arbor, Mich.: Humanities Research Institute, University of Sheffield, Harvester Microform, a former imprint of the Gale Group, and ProQuest Information and Learning Company as part of Early English Books Online (www.oldbaileyonline.org).

N&Q   *Notes and Queries*

W   Ernest Weekley, *Etymological Dictionary of Modern English.* London: John Murray, 1921.

Dedication

v   *ESSE QUAM VIDERI*: From Cicero (*De Amicitia*, 98), means "to be rather than to seem," and was the motto of the Church of England Girls' Grammar School (The Hermitage), now long subsumed into Geelong Grammar School in Corio, Victoria, Australia, but very much alive in the hearts, minds, and example of the Old Girls.

Epigraphs

vii *"Turner's palm"*: J. M. W. Turner (1775–1851); H. J. C. Grierson et al., eds., *The Letters of Sir Walter Scott*, vol. 7, London: Constable & Co., 1934, p. 381.

vii *Balzac*: Page 3; for "filbert" nails see pp. 158–63.

vii *Joyce*: See also Charles T. Dougherty, "Joyce and Ruskin," *N&Q*, February 1953, pp. 76–77, which reveals that the long passage on aesthetics, which Joyce concludes with this sentence, owes much to a comparable passage in John Ruskin's *Fors Clavicera* (1874).

A Note on Finger Numbering and Terminology

xvii Oxford English Dictionary: "finger, *n.*," I. 1. a., vol. 5, pp. 932–35.

xvii *a fifteenth-century source*: Cambridge University Library Manuscript Ff.V.48, lf. 82 (*Catholicon Anglicum*, 131/2). See J. Y. Downing, "A Critical Edition of Cambridge University MS Ff.5.48." Ph.D. dissertation, University of Washington, 1980. Even predating this early document, generations of fearful commentators attributed to each of the five a terrifying array of appropriately chosen vices, beginning with Chaucer in "The Parson's Tale" (borrowing from Peraldus' *Summa de Vitiis et Virtutibus* of 1244–46): "The first finger is the fool looking of the fool woman and of the fool man that sleeth, right as the basilicok sleeth folk by the venom of his sighte: . . . the seconde finger is the vileyns touchinge in wikkede manere. The thridde, is foule words, that fareth lyk fyr that right anon brenneth the herte. The fourthe finger is the kissinge . . . for that mouth is the mouth of helle . . . The fifthe finger of the develes hand is the stinking dede of Lecherie," *cit.* T. M. Pearce, "'Another Knot, Five-Finger-Tied': Shakespeare's 'Troilus and Cressida,' V. ii. 157," *N&Q*, January 1960, pp. 18–19.

xvii *R. W. Burchfield*: Fowler, p. 297.

xviii *Comber*: Thomas Comber, D.D. (1645–99), sometime Precentor of York and Dean of Durham, *cit.* William Jones, F.S.A, *Finger-Ring Lore: Historical, Legendary, Anecdotal*, London: Chatto and Windus, 1890, p. 275, and "the spousal manuals of York and Salisbury," which state of the ring finger, *"quia in illo digito est quaedam vena procedens usque ad cor,"* p. 291.

xviii *Plato: Republic*, Book VII: 523c–d. Edith Hamilton and Huntington Cairns, eds., *The Collected Dialogues of Plato, including the Letters* (Bollingen Series, 71), Princeton, N.J.: Princeton University Press, 1961, p. 755.

xviii *Ness*: London: Printed by T[homas]. Snowdon for the author . . . to be sold by Tho[mas]. Parkhurst . . . , 1690, p. 227, *cit.* Balliolensis, "Death on the Fingers," *N&Q*, 1st series, vol. 8, no. 207, October 15, 1853, p. 362.

xix The Alchemist: I.ii, *cfr.* John Minshew, who runs through the fingers according to which one is suitable for what type of ring: "*Vetus* versiculus singulis digitis annulum *trebuens*, miles, mercator, stultus, maritus, amator. Pollici *ad-*

scribitur militi, *seu* doctori; mercatorum, *à police secundum*; stultorum, tertium, nuptorum vel studiosorum, *quartum*; amatorum, ultimum." See "Ring Finger," *Minshaei Emendatio vel à Mendis Expurgatio seu Augmentatio sui Ductoris in Linguas . . . The Guide to the Tongues . . .*, London: . . . apud Ioannem Browne . . . , 1625, p. 629, *cit.* William Jones, *Finger-Ring Lore*, p. 291 (with numerous errors of transliteration). The passage is translated in *Thaumaturgia, or, Elucidations of the Marvellous*, by an Oxonian (London: Edward Churton, 1835, p. 304): "By which it appears, that the fingers on which annuli [rings] were anciently worn were directed by the calling, or peculiarity of the party. Were it

> A soldier, or doctor, to him was assigned the thumb.
> A sailor, the finger next the thumb.
> A fool, the middle finger.
> A married or diligent person, the fourth or ring finger.
> A lover, the last or little finger."

1. The Finger: A Few Pointers

3 *"How Pleasant to Know Mr. Lear!"*: Edward Lear, *The Complete Verse and Other Nonsense*, edited with an introduction and notes by Vivien Noakes, London and New York: Penguin Books, 2001, p. 428.

3 that *"great bladder for dried peas to rattle in!"*: I am grateful to my teacher and friend Professor Chris Wallace-Crabbe for reminding me of this reference to chapter 6 of *Middlemarch* (1871), which, once noticed, is not easily forgotten, at least not if you work in a large university or, for that matter, an art museum.

4 *colossal marble statue of Emperor Constantine the Great*: See also Anthony Philip Corbeill, *Nature Embodied: Gesture in Ancient Rome*, Princeton: Princeton University Press, 2004, pp. 20–25. *Cfr.* Moshe Barasch, "'Elevatio': The Depiction of a Ritual Gesture," *Artibus et Historiae*, vol. 24, no. 48, 2003, pp. 43–56; Clara Auvray-Assayas, "La main du philosophe," in Philippe Moreau, ed., *Corps romains*, Grenoble: Editions Jérôme Milton, 2002, pp. 15–25, and Mary Beard, "Did Romans Have Elbows?" ibid., pp. 47–59.

6 The Artist Moved to Despair by the Grandeur of Antique Fragments: Zurich: Kunsthaus; Gert Schiff, *Johann Heinrich Füssli, 1741–1825*, Zürich: Verlag Berichthaus, 1973, vol. 1, no. 665, pp. 478–79; Suzanne G. Lindsay, "Emblematic Aspects of Fuseli's Artist in Despair," *Art Bulletin*, vol. 68, no. 3, September 1986, pp. 483–84; Franziska Lentzsch et al., *Fuseli: The Wild Swiss*, Zürich: Verlag Scgeidegger & Speiss, 2005, cat. 1, p. 256.

6 *Sistine Chapel*: Leo Steinberg, "The Line of Fate in Michelangelo's Painting," *Critical Inquiry*, vol. 6, no. 3, Spring 1980, pp. 437–39; Fabrizio Mancinelli, "Michelangelo at Work," in André Chastel, ed., *The Sistine Chapel: Michelangelo Rediscovered*, London: Muller, Blond & White, 1986, pp. 218–59; Wil-

liam E. Wallace, "Michelangelo's Assistants in the Sistine Chapel," *Gazette des Beaux-Arts*, vol. 110, May–June 1987, pp. 203–16; Marcia Hall and Leo Steinberg, "'Who's Who in Michelangelo's *Creation of Adam*' Continued," *Art Bulletin*, vol. 75, no. 2, June 1993, pp. 340–44; Carlo Pietrangeli et al., *The Sistine Chapel: A Glorious Restoration*, New York: Harry N. Abrams, 1994; Maria Rzepinska, "The Divine Wisdom of Michelangelo in *The Creation of Adam*," *Artibus et Historiae*, vol. 15, no. 29, 1994, pp. 181–87; Gosbert Schüßler, "Michelangelos 'Erschaffung des Adam' in der Sixtinischen Kapelle," *Bedeutung in den Bildern: Festschrift für Jörg Traeger zum 60.* Geburtstag (Regensburger Kulturleben, 1), Regensburg: Verlag Schnell & Steiner, 2002, pp. 309–28.

10 The Anatomy of Dr. Nicolaes Tulp: The Hague: Koninklijke Kabinet van Schilderijen, Mauritshuis. See William S. Heckscher, *Rembrandt's Anatomy of Dr. Nicolaes Tulp: An Iconological Study*, New York: New York University Press, 1958, and William Schupbach, *The Paradox of Rembrandt's "Anatomy of Dr. Tulp,"* London: Wellcome Institute for the History of Medicine, 1982, passim (reviewed by David A. Levine in *Art Bulletin*, vol. 68, no. 2, June 1986, pp. 337–40); Dolores Mitchell, "Rembrandt's Anatomy Lesson of Dr. Tulp: A Sinner among the Righteous," *Artibus et Historiae*, vol. 15, no. 30, 1994, pp 145–56.

10 Isenheim Altarpiece: Georg Scheja, *Der Isenheimer Altar des Matthias Grünewald (Matthis Gothart Nithart)*, Cologne: M. DuMont Schauberg, 1969; H. Geissler, B. Saran, J. Harnest, and A. Mischlewski, *Matthis Gothart Nithart, Grünewald: Der Isenheimer Altar*, Stuttgart, 1973; Andrée Hayum, "The Meaning and Function of the Isenheim Altarpiece: The Hospital Context Revisited," *Art Bulletin*, vol. 59, no. 4, December 1977, pp. 501–17; Gottfried Richter, *The Isenheim Altar: Suffering and Salvation in the Art of Grünewald*, translated by Donald Maclean, Edinburgh: Floris, 1998; Franzisca Sarwey, *Grünewald-Studien: zur Realsymbolik des Isenheimer Altars*, herausgegeben und bearbeitet von Harald Möhring, Stuttgart: Urachhaus, 1983. See also Ann Stieglitz, "The Reproduction of Agony: Toward a Reception-History of Grünewald's Isenheim Altar after the First World War," *Oxford Art Journal*, vol. 12, no. 2, 1989, pp. 87–103; Christoph Markschies, "'Hie ist das recht Osterlamm': Christuslamm und Lammsymbolik bei Martin Luther und Lucas Cranach," *Zeitschrift für Kirchengeschichte*, vol. 102, no. 2, 1991, pp 209–30; Willibald Sauerländer, "Mysteries of a Masterpiece," *New York Review of Books*, vol. 38, no. 10, May 30, 1991, pp. 40–42; Diane Apostolos-Cappadona, "The Essence of Agony: Grünewald's Influence on Picasso," *Artibus et Historiae*, vol. 13, no. 26, 1992, pp. 31–47.

12 *caves and other rock shelters*: Miguel Angel García Guinea, *Altamira y los otras cuevas de Cantabria*, 2nd ed., Madrid: Silex Ediciones, 1988; Noel W. Smith, *An Analysis of Ice Age Art, Its Psychology and Belief System* (American University Studies, series 20, Fine Arts, vol. 15), New York: P. Lang, 1992; Groupe de Refléxion sur l'Art Pariétal Paléolithique, *L'Art parietal paléolithique: Techniques et methods*

d'étude (Documents préhistoriques), Paris: Ministère de l'enseignement supérieur et de la recherché, 1993; Christophe Sand et al., "Oceanic Rock Art: First Direct Dating of Prehistoric Stencils and Paintings from New Caledonia (Southern Melanesia)," *Antiquity*, vol. 80, 2006, pp. 523–29.

15 Your Life in Their Hands: BBC Television. Later iterations of this long-running series were shot in color and presented by Jonathan Miller. See Michael Essex-Lopresti, "Your Life in Their Hands," *Lancet*, vol. 368, supplement, December 2006, pp. S24–25.

16 *finger words, expressions, and sayings*: In this section I have obviously relied on *OED*, the *AND*, Fowler, and Partridge, but to those may be added (in chronological order) DA, JCH, F&H, JW, JRW, and W. Also I&M; B&B; HM; Partridge 2; Bozz; A; Burton Stevenson, ed., *The Macmillan Book of Proverbs, Maxims, and Famous Phrases*, New York: The Macmillan Company, 1948; and Jaan Puhvel, "'Finger' in Greek, Latin and Hittite," *Indogermanische Forschungen*, vol. 81, 1976, pp. 25–28.

16 *measurement (a finger's breadth)*: See, for example, T. J. Buckton, "Mediaeval and Modern Measures (2nd S. xi. 328.)," *N&Q*, 2nd series, vol. 11, no. 280, May 11, 1861, p. 376.

16 *resemblance (dead men's fingers)*: A plant, maybe wild orchids, e.g., famously in *Hamlet*, Act IV, sc. vii; see Karl P. Wentersdorf, "*Hamlet*: Ophelia's 'long purples,'" *Shakespeare Quarterly*, vol. 29, 1978, pp. 413–17; Charlotte F. Otten, "Ophelia's 'long purples' or 'dead men's fingers,'" *Shakespeare Quarterly*, vol. 30, 1979, pp. 397–402; and William Hutchings in *Hamlet Studies*, vol. 2, no. 2, 1980, pp. 77–78.

16 *skill (having a green thumb)*: In its current horticultural sense, this expression seems to be comparatively recent. According to the *OED*, the earliest occurrence is in chap. 17 of Robert Carson's novel *Bride Saw Red*, New York: G. P. Putnam's Sons, 1943, p. 203. However, a green thumb of domestic industry, in this case sewing, conspicuously makes it into Louisa May Alcott's *Jack and Jill: A Village Story*, Boston: Roberts Brothers, 1880, chap. 7, p. 78, so the expression seems almost certainly to have a New England provenance.

16 *precision (snapping the fingers)*: See *Manx Sun*, December 22, 1849, p. 6, cit. W. W. G., "Selling a Wife," *N&Q*, vol. 189, pp. 64–65; also J. M. Campbell, "Notes on the Spirit Basis of Belief and Custom," *The Indian Antiquary*, vol. 25, part 316, September 1896, p. 248.

16 *desire (itchy fingers)*: See *The Despatches and Letters of Vice Admiral Lord Viscount Nelson, with Notes, by Sir Nicholas Harris Nicolas*, London: H. Colburn, vol. 2, 1846, p. 280, cit. *OED*, vol. 5, p. 933; satisfactorily, the earliest explicit reference to itchy fingers of desire appears to have been coined in 1796 by Horatio Nelson himself.

16 *concision (thumbnail sketch)*: See Rev. Edward E. Hale, "A Thumb-Nail Sketch," *Sartain's Union Magazine of Literature and Art*, vol. 10, 1852, pp. 39ff., repr. as

"The Old and the New, Face to Face: A Thumb-Nail Sketch" in his *If, Yes, and Perhaps: Four Possibilities and Six Exaggerations, with Some Bits of Fact*, Boston: James R. Osgood & Co., 1876, pp. 100–115.

16 *clumsiness (all thumbs)*: See Anon., "The Busy Bee," *All the Year Round*, n.s., no. 919, Saturday, July 10, 1886, p. 489.

16 *slightness of motion (to stir or lift a finger)*: Matthew 23:4; Luke 11:46.

16 *finger-crossing*: The practice apparently derived from the superstitious belief in the apotropaic effectiveness of making with the index and middle fingers an approximation of the sign of the cross. See B. It remains a vague physical expression of hope for success, or deliverence from calamity, but many other gestures serve a similar purpose, above all various "evil-eye" attitudes such as the Italian *corni* (horns), which are formed by folding over the middle and ring fingers of both hands, and the extension of the index and little fingers.

16 put our finger on it: Or, increasingly rare, *to lay your*, in thought or speculation to fasten onto the exact point (in the midst of surrounding complexity); *cfr. finger on s.o.*, to put the, to point (a wanted man) out to the police (underworld), 20th-cent. U.S. Partridge.

17 at our fingers' ends, *or nowadays at our fingertips*: That is, to be completely familiar with something, derived from the Latin proverb *Scire tanquam ungues digitosque suos*, to which Shakespeare makes reference in *Love's Labour's Lost*, Act V, sc. I: "*Costard*: Got to; thou has it ad dunghill, at the finger's ends, as they say. / *Holofernes*: I smell false Latin; dunghill for unguem." See "finger-end," in "Antedatings from Nicholas Udall's Translation of Erasmus's 'Apophthegmes,'" *N&Q*, December 1967, p. 447. By contrast, the *OED* cites the earliest occurrence of *fingertips* (in the plural) as Alfred Tennyson's "Sir Launcelot and Queen Guinevere" (1842): "As fast as she fled thro' sun and shade, / The happy winds upon her play'd, / Blowing the ringlet from the braid: / She look'd so lovely, as she sway'd / The rein with dainty finger-tips, / A man had given all other bliss, / And all his worldly worth for this, / To waste his whole heart in one kiss / Upon her perfect lips," and it may well be that *fingers' ends* was replaced by the current term *fingertips* as a direct result of Tennyson's rhyme scheme.

17 *"an admirable finger upon the harpsichord"*: cit. *OED*.

17 *George Arliss*: Gerald Lawrence, rev. K. D. Reynolds, *ODNB*, vol. 2, p. 390. On January 14, 1687, James Audley was tried at the Old Bailey for uttering seditious words, namely "that Monmouth had more honesty in his little Finger, than the King had in his whole Body, &c." He was acquitted when it was found that the prosecution was malicious. *POB* t16870114–29.

17 *"my little finger shall be thicker than my father's loins"*: 2 Chronicles 10:10. See Francesco Vattioni, "3 (1) Re 12, 10; Par (Cr) 10, 10 e Teodoreto di Ciro," *Augustinianum*, vol. 31, 1991, pp. 475–77, where a better translation (via Syriac) is proposed: "My little finger is larger than my father's thumb." However, the

little finger/father's loins image endured powerfully, and crops up often in seventeenth-century England, for example in *Articles of Impeachment Exhibited Against Col. Robert Gibbons and Cap. Richard Yeardley, Late Governors of the Isle of Jersey . . . Wherein the several impeachments, actions, high misdemeanours . . . are laid open . . . as also a remedy for the people against the heavy yoke of such tyrannical oppressours in this juncture of miraculous restauration after so long a bondage, wherein the little finger of some appeared heavier then* [sic] *the whole loins of others*, London: Printed for G. Horton, 1659.

17 *"Thy hand is but a finger to my fist"*: *King Henry VI, Part II*, Act IV, sc. x.

17 Troilus and Cressida: Act V, sc. ii.

17 *Aristotle*: Cynthia Freeland, "Aristotle on the Sense of Touch," in Martha C. Nussbaum and Amélie Oksenberg Rorty, eds., *Essays on Aristotle's* De Anima, Oxford: Oxford University Press (The Clarendon Press), 1992, pp. 227–48.

19 to put the finger in your eye: See *The Comedy of Errors*, Act II, sc. ii: "Come, come, no longer will I be a fool, / To put the finger in the eye and weep." See also George Cheatham, "Shakespeare's *The Taming of the Shrew*," *Explicator*, vol. 42, no. 3, 1984, p. 12; noting the sense in Act I, sc. i, where Katherine says of Bianca ". . . it is best to put the finger in the eye, and she knew not why."

19 *a wet finger*: Or *wet finger, with a*, obs., easily, smoothly, or directly, possibly derived from the craft of spinning wool: the fibers are more easily regulated when the spinner keeps the forefinger wet with saliva (e.g., Anon., *The Wisdome of Doctor Dodypoll*, 1600: "*Flores*: Canst thou bring me thither? *Peasant*: With a wet finger"), but it may alternatively be a nautical reference: Sailors may determine the direction of the wind by holding up a wetted finger. B. See also F. C. Birkbeck Terry, "William Gouge's 'Whole-Armor of God,' 1616: 'With a Wet Finger' (6th S. xi. 222)," *N&Q*, 6th series, vol. 11, April 25, 1885, pp. 331–32.

19 *to be* under someone's thumb: See Charles Dickens's *David Copperfield* (1850), chap. xxv: ". . . under his thumb. Un—der—his thumb," said Uriah, very slowly, as he stretched out his cruel-looking hand above my table, and pressed his own thumb down upon it, until it shook, and shook the room."

19 having a finger in every pie: See *King Henry VIII*, Act I, sc. i: "*Buckingham*: The devil speed him! no man's pie is freed / From his ambitious finger."

19 finger trouble: "He's lazy; he is given to procrastination," R.A.F., since c. 1935; also *to have the finger up* or *to have the finger well in*, "mostly Army, from 1940 onwards." Partridge. *Cfr. finger trouble*, coll., an error, possibly habitual, caused by pressing the wrong keys or buttons of an electric machine. B3 (unattrib.).

19 to put the finger on someone: to point (a wanted man) out to the police (underworld), 20th-cent. U.S. Partridge.

19 getting your fingers burned *or* scorched (*that is, snuffing out another man's candle*): To experience a harmful mishap; also said to be derived from picking roasted chestnuts out of the fire. B.

19 caught in the till: To be caught red-handed stealing from your employer. B3
thinks that this "expression is open to elaboration as required," citing *The
Times*, February 27, 1999: "[the Right Hon. Peter] Lilley [Conservative M.P.
for Hitchen and Harpenden] was not so much fired from the Shadow Cabi-
net but [*sic*] chucked out like some shop assistant caught with both hands,
both legs and several other body parts in the till."

19 light-fingered: U.K., since the 1950s. B2.

19 fingers made of lime twigs: That is, a thief, late 16th to 18th cent., coll. Har-
ington, 1596; Bailey 1739; Apperson. Partridge.

19 each finger was a fish hook: As in evidence given by one Nicholas Huggin-
son at the Old Bailey in London in the trial of Francis Skinner and others for
theft and simple grand larceny, October 15, 1729, *POB*, t17291015–73.

19 letting something slip through your fingers: To miss an opportunity, possibly
derived from cricket, as in a dropped catch, or else nautical, as in a slipped
sheet or rope.

20 Getting your fingers inked: See Lady Mary Wortley Montagu to Lady Rich,
March 16, 1718, *Complete Letters of Lady Mary Wortley Montagu*, edited by
Robert Halsband, Oxford: Oxford University Press (The Clarendon Press),
vol. 1, 1965, p. 389. Previously, however, the expression was used far less
literally. For example, in 1562 James Pilkington, Bishop of Durham, in the
preface to his "Exposition Vpon Abdyas [Obediah]," remarked of his sectarian
enemies: "But alas for pity! for lack of sharp discipline they lie lurking and
looking for that day when they may turn to their old vomit again, enking
[inking] their hands in blood . . ." *The Works of James Pilkington* . . . , edited for
the Parker Society by the Rev. James Scholefield, Cambridge: Cambridge
University Press, 1842, p. 211.

20 finger-wagging: N.B., however, that the *OED* makes it clear that in English,
the action of wagging reached the fingers only comparatively recently, having
for centuries worked its way down from the head, via whole limbs, and the
tongue.

20 finger-pointing: See G. A. Starr in *N&Q*, December 1967, p. 444, where the
phrase is traced to *Apophthegmes, that is to saie, prompte, quicke, wittie and senten-
tious saiynges* (London: Richard Grafton, 1542), predating the earliest reference in *OED*.

20 giving somebody the finger: See pp. 192–206.

20 a bit for the finger: "an extremely intimate caress, the recipient being a
woman," 19th-cent., low. Partridge.

20 well-thumbed: *Cfr. thumb*, v., 1. to handle, paw (*OED*); 2. to read and re-read
either desultorily (e.g., magazines) or, at times also, studiously (e.g., well-
thumbed prayerbook); 3. "to drain (a glass) upon a thumb-nail"; 4. "to possess
(a woman)," 18th to 19th cent., lingering into the first decade of the 20th
cent. as *well-thumbed (girl)*, "'a foundered whore'" (F&H); 5. to ask a passing
motorist for a free ride, from c. 1940.

20 finger-and-thumb: n., 1. a road (underworld) rhyming on Gypsy *drum*, late 19th to 20th cent.; 2. rum, rhyming slang (J. C. H.; H. M., vol. 1; D. A., 1857, as *finger-thumb*); 3. "A companion or mate," rhyming slang, with *chum*, since c. 1930; "term of contempt for man or woman" (underworld, via the ex-burglar George Ingram [I.&M.], 1930).

20 *a racketeer's cut of exactly 10 percent*: Partridge 2.

21 busmen's finger: [hence?] an official, i.e., "busmen's finger," c. 1930, *Daily Herald*, August 5, 1930, n.p. Partridge. See also A.E.B. and Edmund Tew, " 'The Finger of Scorn' (5th S. iii. 39, 154.)," *N&Q*, 5th series, vol. 3, May 15, 1875, p. 397.

21 fingerpost: n., 1. "A post set up at the parting of roads, with one or more arms [*sic*], often terminating in the shape of a finger, to indicate the directions of the several roads; a guide-post" (*OED*, 1789) [see also *finger-board*], hence *finger-posted*, ppl. a., and *finger-postless*; 2. fig., "a parson, so called, because like the finger post, he points out a way he . . . probably will never go, *i.e.*, the way to heaven" (1785) *OED*.

21 fingers *of a clock*: See also *King Richard II*, where this usage creeps into Richard's speech about time in Act V, sc. v: "I wasted time, and now doth time waste me; / For now hath time made me his numbering clock: / My thoughts are minutes; and with sighs they jar / Their watches unto mine eyes, the outward watch, / whereto my finger, like a dial's point, / Is pointing still, in cleansing them from tears."

21 *numbers to the power of ten*: See pp. 95–104.

21 *finger bowls*: F. Bradbury, "Finger-Bowls (clxiii. 350)," *N&Q*, November 26, 1932, p. 390.

22 *winningly dimpled knuckles*: When in Marivaux's play *Jeu de l'amour et du hazard* (1730), about to take Lisette's hand in marriage, the character of Arlequin describes it affectionately as *"rondelette et potelée"* (strictly speaking, the equivalent of "pottled," meaning plump, but surely also implying the presence of dimples), he could be describing exactly the hand of a Boucher shepherdess. I am grateful to my senior colleague Claude Rawson for offering me this useful reference.

22 *Velázquez*: See, for example, Aureliano de Beruete, *Velazquez*, translated by Hugh E. Poynter, London: Methuen and Co., 1906, p. 121, but similar observations are made constantly throughout the literature.

22 *van Dyck's astonishing way with gloves*: See p. 122.

22 *"filbert" nails*: See pp. 158–63.

22 *glove trade*: See pp. 117–46.

22 Guernica: Susan Grace Galassi, "The Arnheim Connection: *Guernica* and *Las Meninas*," *Journal of Aesthetic Education*, vol. 27, no. 4, Winter 1993, pp. 45–56; Kathleen Brunner, 'Guernica': The Apocalypse of Representation," *Burlington Magazine*, vol. 143, no. 1175, February 2001, pp. 80–85.

26 *Giovanni Morelli*: At first Morelli wrote under the curious part-anagrammatic, part-pseudonymous split personality of Ivan Lermolieff (a putatively Russian

author) and Johannes Schwarze (his German translator). See Jaynie Anderson, "Morelli's Scientific Method of Attribution; Origins and Interpretations," in H. Olbrich, ed., *L'Art et les révolutions: Actes [du] XXVIIe Congrès international d'histoire de l'art, Strasbourg, 1–7 septembre 1989*, Strasbourg: Société alsacienne pour le développement de l'histoire de l'art, 1992, pp. 135–41; David Carrier, "Winckelmann and Pater, Morelli and Freud: The Tropics of Art Historical Discourse," *History of the Human Sciences*, vol. 2, 1989, pp. 19–38; Carol Gibson-Wood, "Art History and Connoisseurship at the Beginning of the Nineteenth Century" and "Giovanni Morelli," sections IV and V of her *Studies in the Theory of Connoisseurship from Vasari to Morelli*, New York and London: Garland, 1988, pp. 138–65, 169–247; Hayden B. J. Maginnis, "The Role of Perceptual Learning in Connoisseurship: Morelli, Berenson and Beyond," *Art History*, vol. 13, March 1990, pp. 104–17; J. J. Spector, "The Method of Morelli and Its Relation to Freudian Psychoanalysis," in *Diogenes*, no. 66, Summer 1969, pp. 63–83; Richard Wollheim, "Giovanni Morelli and the Origins of Scientific Connoisseurship," chap. 9 of his *On Art and the Mind*, London: Allen Lane, 1973, pp. 177–201; Carlo Ginzburg, "Morelli, Freud, and Sherlock Holmes: Clues and Scientific Method," *History Workshop: A Journal of Socialist Historians*, vol. 9, 1980, pp. 5–36 (reprinted as "Clues: Morelli, Freud, and Sherlock Holmes," in Umberto Eco and Thomas Albert Sebeok, eds., *The Sign of Three: Dupin, Holmes, Peirce*, Bloomington: Indiana University Press, 1983, pp. 81–118). But see also the important recent critique by Mary D. Garrard, "Artemisia's Hand," chap. 3 of Norma Broude and Mary D. Garrard, eds., *Reclaiming Female Agency: Feminist Art History after Postmodernism*, Berkeley, Calif.: University of California Press, 2005, pp. 63–78.

2. The Finger and the Hand

As will become clear, in much of this chapter I have relied on Henry Gray's *Anatomy, Descriptive and Surgical*, in the revised American edition (which is based on the 15th English edition), New York: Gramercy Books, 1977, and on the following medical texts, which I list in chronological order: Johan Matthijs Frederick Landsmeer, *Anatomical and Functional Investigations on the Articulation of the Human Fingers*, Basel and New York: S. Karger, 1955; Lee W. Milford, *Retaining Ligaments of the Digits of the Hand: Gross and Microscopic Anatomical Study*, Philadelphia: W. B. Saunders and Co., 1968; Emanuel B. Kaplan, *Functional and Surgical Anatomy of the Hand*, 3rd ed. Philadelphia: Lippincott, 1984; Graham Lister, *The Hand: Diagnosis and Indications*, 2nd ed., Edinburgh, etc.: Churchill Livingstone, 1984; John Napier, *Hands* (edited by Russell H. Tuttle), Princeton: Princeton University Press, 1993; James Steven Hovius et al., eds., *The Pediatric Upper Limb*, London: Martin Dunitz, 2002; and Lynette A. Jones and Susan J. Lederman, *Human Hand Function*, New York: Oxford University Press, 2006. I have endeavored to check and double-check the medical facts for accuracy, and have also benefited from the extremely generous remedial scientific advice and assistance of my old friend Dr. Adam Jenney, of the Alfred Hospital in Melbourne.

31 *Montaigne*: "Apologie de Raimond de Sebonde," *Essais*, II:xii, translated by John Florio, London: printed by V. Sims for E. Blount, 1603. The original text: *"Quoy des mains? Nous requerons, nous promettons, appellons, congedions, menaçons, prions, supplions, nions, refusons, interrogeons, admirons, nombrons, confessons, repentons, craignons, vergoignons, doubtons, instruisons, commandons, incitons, encourageons, jurons, tesmoignons, accusons, condamnons, absolvons, injurions, mesprisons, deffions, despittons, flattons, applaudissons, benissons, humilions, moquons, reconcilions, recommandons, exaltons, festoyons, resjouïssons, complaignons, attristons, desconfortons, desesperons, estonnons, escrions, taisons: et quoy non? d'une variation et multiplication à l'envy de la langue."*

35 *third phalanx in the thumb*: In fact, this abnormality can and does occur in what has been estimated at one in 25,000 live births, and amazing pediatric hand surgeons can successfully remove the extra phalanx before it causes developmental havoc. See Steven E. R. Hovius, J. Michiel Zuidam, and Thijs de Wit, "Treatment of the Triphalangeal Thumb," *Techniques in Hand and Upper Extremity Surgery*, vol. 8, no. 4, December 2004, pp. 247–56.

44 Proceedings of the Old Bailey: On September 10, 1680, three men were tried for the murder of Robert Stanly, Esq., whose finger was cut in a scuffle in King Street, London (*POB*, t16800910a-1).

45 *"Edling"*: *POB*, t16820712-9. In 1695, the widow Parthenia Owen of the Parish of St. Giles's in the Fields was acquitted of the murder of her husband, George, the first joint of whose middle finger she claimed she bit, bruised, and dislocated "by accident" in the course of a domestic quarrel. Gangrene gradually crept all the way up to Mr. Owen's shoulder, and he died four months later (*POB*, t16950508-12).

45 *Mrs. Billington*: *The Times*, March 25, 1790, p. 2.

45 *Lady Maria Wentworth*: J. L. (Royal Dublin Society), "Death from Wounding the Finger with a Needle," *N&Q*, 3rd series, vol. 2, August 30, 1862, p. 173.

45 *Duke of Queensberry*: 1724–1810 (the fourth in the peerage of Scotland, where no doubt the climate did little to assist in His Grace's recovery. *The Times*, January 2, 1802, p. 3.

45 *law columns*: Simmons v. Great Northern Railway Company, *Reynolds's Newspaper*, Sunday, August 12, 1866, p. 8, and "Metropolitan Railway Company v. Jackson," *Illustrated Police News*, December 22, 1877, p. 3. The plaintiff in the second case was unlucky that his vain and costly quest for just compensation straddled the passing of the Supreme Court of Judicature Acts (36 & 37 Victoria chap. 66 and 38 & 39 Victoria chap. 77), which expensively rearranged most avenues of litigation in England.

46 *Hox genes*: Clifford J. Tabin, "Why We Have (Only) Five Fingers Per Hand: Hox Genes and the Evolution of Paired Limbs," *Development*, 116, 1992, pp. 289–96; Denis Duboule, ed., *Guidebook to the Homeobox Genes*, Oxford: Oxford

University Press, 1994; Walter J. Gehring, *Master Control Genes in Development and Evolution: The Homeobox Story*, New Haven: Yale University Press, 1998; Frances R. Goodman, "Mutations in the Human *HOX* Genes," in S. Malcolm and J. Goodship, eds., *Genotype to Phenotype*, 2nd ed., Oxford: BIOS Scientific Publishers, 2001, pp. 209–27; Malcolm Logan, "Finger or Toe: The Molecular Basis of Limb Identity," *Development*, 130, 2003, pp. 6401–10; John Cobb and Denis Duboule, "Comparative Analysis of Genes Downstream of the Hoxd Cluster in Developing Digits and External Genitalia," *Development*, 132, 2005, pp. 3055–67; Spyros Papageorgiou, ed., *Hox Gene Expression*, New York: Springer Science and Business Media, 2007.

48 *one bone, followed by two bones, followed by a collection of small, bloblike bones*: Neil Shubin, *Your Inner Fish: A Journey into the 3.5-Billion-Year History of the Human Body*, New York: Random House, 2008, p. 31.

3. The Finger of God

51 *Exodus 31:18*: King James; the Vulgate reads *"dedit quoque Mosi conpletis huiuscemodi sermonibus in monte Sinai duas tabulas testimonii lapideas scriptas* digito Dei."

51 *Sanjūsangendō*: Emily Joy Sano, "The Twenty-Eight Bushū of Sanjūsangendō," Columbia University Ph.D. dissertation, 1983.

52 *Albert E. Elsen*: "Images of Gods," in Carole Gold Calo, ed., *Writings about Art*, Englewood Cliffs, N.J.: Prentice Hall, 1994, p. 11, an extract from his *Purposes of Art: An Introduction to the History and Appreciation of Art*, 4th ed., New York: Holt, Rinehart and Winston, 1974, p. 39.

52 *gestures of benediction*: Martin Kirigin, O.S.B., *La mano divina nell'iconografia cristiana* (Studi di antichità cristiana, 31), Rome: Pontificia Istituto di Archeologia Cristiana, 1976, p. 213; Howard Jacobson, "The Position of the Fingers during the Priestly Blessing," *Revue de Qumran*, vol. 34, 1977, pp. 259–60.

58 *Isaiah*: 11:3–4.

59 *discrete fingers are mentioned far less often but quite strategically*: See, for example, Anna Maria Schwemer, "Gottes Hand und die Propheten: Zum Wandel der Metapher 'Hand Gottes' in frühjüdischer Zeit," in René Kieffer et Jan Bergman, eds., *La Main de Dieu = Die Hand Gottes* (Wissenschaftliche Untersuchungen zum Neuen Testament, 94), Tübingen: J. C. B. Mohr (Paul Siebeck), 1997, pp. 65–85; Scott B. Noegel, "Moses and Magic: Notes on the Book of Exodus," *Journal of the Ancient Near Eastern Society*, vol. 24, 1996, pp. 45–59.

61 *"many" Greek and Latin manuscripts [of John]*: The hundred-year literature on the *pericope adulterae* is enormous, and illustrates the extent of the late-nineteenth- and twentieth-century fixation on the sinister idea of adulteresses and adultery in general. The most convenient recent porthole is Jennifer Wright Knust's long article "Early Christian Re-Writing and the History of

the *Pericope Adulterae*," *Journal of Early Christian Studies*, vol. 14, no. 4, 2006, pp. 485–536, upon which I have relied for much of what follows.

62 the pericope adulterae *definitely belongs in John*: Bart D. Ehrman, "Jesus and the Adulteress," *New Testament Studies*, vol. 34, 1988, pp. 24–25.

63 the measure *of symbolic intensity*: Raymond E. Brown, *The Gospel according to John, I–XII* (The Anchor Bible, 29), New York: Doubleday, 1966, p. 336; Andrew McGowan, personal communication with the author, April 11, 2007.

63 draws *lines, or "doodles in the dust"*: Brown, *John*, p. 334, *cit*. Knust, n. 97, p. 514. Also W. Alfred Tisdale, Jr., personal communication with the author, April 10, 2007.

63 "*Jesus' finger is the finger of God writing the law, as in Exodus*": Andrew McGowan, personal communication with the author, April 11, 2007; but see also T. J. Buckton, "Writing on the Ground," *N&Q*, 3rd series, vol. 12, August 24, 1867, pp. 145–46; A. Nugent, "What Did Jesus Write? (John 7, 53–8, 11)," *Downside Review*, vol. 108, no. 372, 1990, pp. 193–98; Harald Schöndorf, "Jesus schreibt mit dem Finger auf die Erde: Joh 8:6 b. 8," *Biblische Zeitschrift*, vol. 40, no. 1, 1996, pp. 91–93.

64 an increasingly *"anti-Jewish" early Christian standpoint*: This is the thrust of Knust's argument, pp. 532–36.

64 esoteric *iconographical tradition*: See also G. T. R., "Anachronisms of Painters," *N&Q*, June 28, 1851, p. 517, who recorded an example by Hendrik van Steenwyk (1550–1603) "in which our Lord is made to write in *Dutch!*"; B. H. C., "Anachronisms of Painters," ibid., November 8, 1851, pp. 369–70, who defended that usage and mentioned that he knew many instances of the inscription given in Latin, and W. T., ibid., 5th series, vol. 6, August 26, 1876, p. 169, who recorded what is presumably a relatively early, apparently sixteenth-century example in English from Lincolnshire. "Lysart" (ibid., 7th series, vol. 2, December 11, 1886, p. 474) claimed to have located a reference to "Gautama Sakyamuni," the Buddha, having performed arithmetical calculations "with the 'finger on sand,'" though it is unclear what conclusion he proposed to draw from that, other than that the practice appears to have been vaguely associated with holiness. A more pertinent observation from J. J. Fahie followed in vol. 3, April 30, 1887, p. 358, to the effect that Turkomen women had been observed tracing the pattern for carpets in sand, implying a Near Eastern and/or Central Asian continuity. That George Noble's renewed query about John 8:6 (7th series, vol. 2, November 6, 1886, apparently prompted by Lingard's *New Version of the Four Gospels* [1836]) generated so much discussion in *N&Q* at this date is no doubt due to the widespread fascination with biblical archaeology, which had been hugely enhanced by the publication in 1849 of Layard's *Nineveh*.

66 Numerous *other patristic commentators of the fourth century*: Brown, *John*, p. 334, but see also Brad H. Young, "'Save the Adulteress!' Ancient Jewish *Responsa*

in the Gospels?" *New Testament Studies*, vol. 41, 1995, p. 69, where "writing *halachah* (the law, *i.e.* in this case judgment) was forbidden" and "if what Jesus wrote in the dirt was so integral to the resolution of the conflict, the exact words would have been recorded in the narrative." See also the following fascinating exchange stemming from George Noble's "Writing on Sand," *N&Q*, 7th series, vol. 2, November 6, 1886, p. 369; "Lysart," and M. Damant, December 11, 1886, p. 474; S. J. Chadwick, vol. 3, January 8, 1887, p. 36; J. J. Fahie, vol. 3, March 19, 1887, p. 231, and April 30, 1887, p. 358; "St. Swithin," vol. 6, September 22, 1888, p. 236; T. Adolphus Trollope, W. C. B., and R. H. Busk, vol. 6, November 6, 1888, p. 369.

67 *Didymus' précis*: Ehrman, p. 32, *cit.* Ulrich Becker, *Jesus und die Ehebrecherin* (Berlin: Alfred Topelmann, 1963), pp. 82–91.

67 *he was certainly learned*: André Lemaire, "Writing and Writing Materials," in David Noel Freedman et al., eds., *The Anchor Bible Dictionary*, vol. VI, New York: Doubleday, 1992, p. 1005.

68 *early-first-century Palestine*: Dale Martin, personal communication with the author, July 6, 2007.

68 *slow country bumpkins*: Geza Vermes, *The Changing Face of Jesus*, New York: Viking Compass, 2001, pp. 243–46.

69 *a prominent local family, that of M—— (in ——shire)*: Anon., "The Angel's Finger," *Trewman's Exeter Flying Post*, December 21, 1864, p. 6. The author goes on to report that the phenomenon had occurred again lately, but this time presaged the murder of several relations at Meerut and Delhi during the Indian Mutiny of 1857–58.

71 *Mudras*: The literature is truly vast, but I have benefited especially from Ananda Kentish Coomaraswamy and Gopala Kristnayya Duggirala, *The Mirror of Gesture*, New Delhi: Munshiram Manoharlal Publishers, 1997 (a valuable English translation of the second-century C.E. Abhinaya-Darpana by Nandikeshvara. The Abhinaya-Darpana is an abridgement of the Bharatarnava, an exposition on the art of Indian dancing); E. Dale Saunders, *Mudrā: A Study of Symbolic Gestures in Japanese Buddhist Sculpture*, Princeton, N.J.: Princeton University Press, 1960; Gosta Liebert, *Iconographic Dictionary of the Indian Religions, Hinduism, Buddhism, Jainism*, Leyden: Brill, 1976; Lokesh Chandra and Sharada Rani, *Mudras in Japan: Symbolic Hand-Postures in Japanese Mantrayana or the Esoteric Buddhism of the Shingon Denomination* (Sata-Pikata Series, 243), New Delhi: Sata-Pikata, 1978; O. Frankfurter, "The Attitudes of the Buddha," *Journal of the Siam Society*, vol. 10, no. 2, 1913, pp. 1–36; Ramesh S. Gupte, *Iconography of the Hindus, Buddhists and Jains*, Bombay (Mumbai): D. B. Taraporevala Sons and Co., 1972; T. A. Gopinatha Rao, *Elements of Hindu Iconography*, Madras (Chennai): The Law Printing House, 1914; and Fredrick W. Bunce, *Mudrās in Buddhist and Hindu Practice: An Iconographic Consideration*, New Delhi: D. K. Printworld, 2001.

72 *Monier Monier-Williams*: *Hinduism*, London: Society for Promoting Christian Knowledge, New York: Pott, Young, 1877, p. 127.
72 *Bunce*: *Mūdras in Buddhist and Hindu Practice*, pp. xxvi–xxvii.
74 *Thai representations of the postures of the Lord Buddha*: Ibid., pp. 324–26.
74 dharmachakra *mudra:* Ibid., p. 58, fig. 139.
75 nalini-padmakosha *mudra:* Ibid., p. 148, fig. 360.
75 kamjayi *mudra:* Ibid., p. 100, fig. 234.
75 bhumisparsha *mudra*: Ibid., pp. 33–34, fig. 78.

4. The Finger and Communication

77 *Bacon*: *Essay LVI: Of Iudicature* (1625), for which see *Bacon's Essays*, edited by Alfred S. West, Cambridge: Cambridge University Press, 1908, p. 167, and note 3, where it is made clear that "ancient" meant not old but senior.
77 *pointing*: George Butterworth, "Pointing Is the Royal Road to Language for Babies," chap. 2 of Sotaro Kita, ed., *Pointing: Where Language, Culture, and Cognition Meet*, Mahwah, N.J., and London: Lawrence Erlbaum Associates, 2003, pp. 8–33; Danielle Bouvet, "L'Approche des configurations de la main dans les langues gestuelles selon des critères articulatoires," *La Main* (Eurasie: Cahiers de la Société des Études euro-asiatiques, 4), Paris: Editions L'Harmattan, 1993, pp. 27–44; D. Givens, "The Big and the Small: Toward a Paleontology of Gesture," *Sign Language Studies*, vol. 51, 1986, pp. 145–70; Mary E. Hazard, *Elizabethan Silent Language*, Lincoln: University of Nebraska Press, 2000; William C. Stokoe, *Language in Hand: Why Sign Came before Speech*, Washington, D.C.: Gallaudet University Press, 2001.
80 *"biologically based, and species specific"*: Stokoe, *Language in Hand*, pp. 28–29.
80 *cultural history of gesture*: In this section I have relied above all upon C. Chambers and K. Craig, "Similarities and Differences between Cultures in Expressive Movements," in Hinde, R., ed., *Non-Verbal Communication*, Cambridge: Cambridge University Press, 1972, pp. 297–314; Jan Bremmer and Herman Roodenburg, eds., *A Cultural History of Gesture*, Ithaca, NY: Cornell University Press, 1992; David McNeill, *Hand and Mind: What Gestures Reveal about Thought*, Chicago: Chicago University Press, 1992; Jean-Hubert Levame, "Main-objet et main-image," in *La Main* (Eurasie: Cahiers de la Société des Études euro-asiatiques, 4), Paris: Editions L'Harmattan, 1993, pp. 9–18; Philippe Seringe, "Symbolisme de la main," ibid., pp. 45–54; Betty J. Bäuml and Franz H. Bäuml, *Dictionary of Worldwide Gestures*, 2nd ed., Lanham, Md., and London: Scarecrow Press, 1997; and Tiziana Baldizzone et al., *La Main qui parle*, Paris: Phébus, 2002.
80 *Italy*: Bruno Munari, *Supplemento al dizionario italiano*, 2nd ed. Mantua: Maurizio Corraini Editore, 2007, pp. 22, 26, 60, 106.
84 *Prayer and benediction; magic and incantation*: See Jean Umiker-Sebeok and Thomas A. Sebeok, "Sign Languages: The Problem of Classification," in their

Monastic Sign Languages (Approaches to Semiotics, vol. 76), Berlin, Amsterdam, and New York: Mouton de Gruyter & Co., 1987, pp. viii–xiii; Robert A. Barakat, *The Cistercian Sign Language: A Study in Non-Verbal Communication*, Kalamazoo, Mich.: Cistercian Publications, 1975.

85 "*different sorts of bread . . . 'as well'*": Dom Louis Gougard, "Le Langage des silencieux," chap. 2 of his *Anciennes coutumes claustrales*, Ligugé: Abbeye Saint-Martin de Ligugé, 1930, pp. 95–96, *cit*. Robert A. Barakat, "Cistercian Sign Language," in Umiker-Sebeok and Sebeok, *Monastic Sign Languages*, p. 89 (*"les différentes sortes de pains; les legumes, les poisons, les fruits, les autres comestibles, les aromates, les liquids, les vases, les vêtements, les objets liturgiques, les choses relatives à la celebration de la messe et de l'office divin, les vêtements liturgiques, les livres usuels, les différentes sortes de personnes, d'édifices, d'instruments et d'outils et d'autres choses encore"*).

86 *fake signs*: Barakat in Umiker-Sebeok and Sebeok, *cit*. Gérard van Rijnberk, *Le Langage par signes chez les moines*, Amsterdam: Koninklijke Nederlandse Academie van Wetenschappen, Noordhollandse Uitgeverij, 1953, p. 11.

86 *riotous commotion*: Barakat in Umiker-Sebeok and Sebeok, *cit*. Eva Matthews Sanford, "De Loquela Digitorum," *Classical Journal*, vol. 23, no. 8, May 1928, p. 593.

87 *abbé de l'Épée: L'Institution des sourds et muets par la voie des signes méthodiques: ouvrage qui contient le project d'une langue universelle, par l'entremise des signes naturels assujettis à une méthode*, Paris: Chez Nyon l'aîné, 1776. See also Freeman G. Henry, *Language, Culture, and Hegemony in Modern France (1533 to the Millennium)*, Birmingham, Ala.: Summa Publications, 2008, sections 4.3.1.–4.3.4., pp. 115–22; Maryse Bézagu-Deluy, *L'Abbé de l'Epée: instituteur gratuit des sourds et muets, 1712–1789*, Paris: Seghers, 1990; Renate Fischer and Harlan Lane, eds., *Looking Back: A Reader on the History of Deaf Communities and Their Sign Languages* (International Studies on Sign Language and Communication of the Deaf, 20), Hamburg: Signum Verlag, 1993; Cecil Lucas, ed., *Pinky Extension and Eye Gaze: Language Use in Deaf Communities* (Sociolinguistics in Deaf Communities series, 4), Washington, D.C.: Gallaudet University Press, 1998; Cecil Lucas, ed., *Turn-Taking, Fingerspelling and Contact in Signed Languages*, Washington, D.C.: Gallaudet University Press, 2002.

88 *five distinct types of gestures*: Barakat in Umiker-Sebeok and Sebeok, pp. 99–112.

89 *American Sign Language*: Fischer and Lane, pp. 25–30.

90 *kanji, hiragana, katakana, and romaji*: Christopher Seeley, *A History of Writing in Japan*, Honolulu: University of Hawai'i Press, 1991, pp. 70ff.

90 *Braille*: Jean Roblin, *Les Doigts qui lisent: vie de Louis Braille, 1809–1852*, with a preface by Georges Bidault. Monte Carlo: Regain, 1951.

91 *not the first form of writing for the blind*: James Wilson, *Biography of the Blind: Including the Lives of All Who Have Distinguished Themselves as Poets, Philosophers, Artists, &c., &c.*, collected and edited by Keneth A. Stuckey from the four original editions of 1821–38. Washington, D.C.: Library of Congress, 1995.

91 *Mademoiselle de Salignac*: Ibid., pp. 268–73.

92 *manicule*: William H. Sherman, "Towards a History of the Manicule," chap. 2 of his *Used Books: Marking Readers in Renaissance England*, Philadelphia: University of Pennsylvania Press, 2008, pp. 25–52.

92 *American Typefounders Company*: Charles Hasler, "A Show of Hands," *Typographica*, o.s., vol. 8, 1953, pp. 4–11.

5. The Finger and the Economy

95 *"She shows that wives are wont to be selected"*: St. Jerome, on Roman women in general and in particular on Marcia, the virtuous younger daughter of Cato, *Adversus Jovinianum*, I:46: *"multos non oculis sed* digitis *uxores ducere"* (my italics).

95 *system of numbering to the power of ten*: See Karl Menninger, "Numbering by Fingers and Toes," in his *Number Words and Number Symbols: A Cultural History of Numbers*, translated by Paul Broneer, Cambridge, Mass.: MIT Press, 1969, pp. 35–38. See also H. Campbell, "Octaval Notation," *N&Q*, February 15, 1930, p. 113.

95 *the joints of four fingers minus the thumb*: Vasili Sinaïski, *Counting as Primordial Base of Human Culture (New Methodology)* (Epistolae et Logistorici, 15–18), Riga, Latvia: Ed. "Aequitas," 1933, p. 14.

95 *First Nations Americans*: John D. Barrow, *The Book of Nothing*, London: Jonathan Cape, 2000, p. 15, citing his own *Pi in the Sky*, Oxford: Oxford University Press, 1992.

96 *Henry Attwell*: "'Thirty Days Hath September' (8th S. iii. 245, 475; iv. 77, 337)," *N&Q*, 8th series, vol. 5, May 12, 1894, pp. 373–74.

98 *late Regency Shropshire and Cheshire*: B. Smith, "Toe and Finger Names," *N&Q*, 11th series, vol. 2, September 10, 1910, p. 217.

98 *"Tom Thumbkin"*: E. P., "Counting on Fingers (clxxxiv, 49, 147, 205)," *N&Q*, April 10, 1943, p. 239.

98 *worrying Nottinghamshire version*: Thomas Ratcliffe of Worksop, ibid.

99 *"Thumb, Black Barney"*: Charlemont, "Counting on Fingers," *N&Q*, January 16, 1943, p. 48. See also M. H. Dodds, "Counting on Fingers," *N&Q*, March 27, 1943, p. 205, who proposes that "Black Barney loups the dyke, steals the corn, runs away, and Little Canny Wanny [who has nothing to do with it] pays for all."

99 *"This is the man who broke the barn"* and *"This broke the barn"*: J. D. Hutchison, "Counting on Fingers (clxxxiv, 48)," *N&Q*, February 27, 1943, p. 147. See also James Orchard Halliwell-Phillips, *Popular Rhymes and Nursery Tales*, London: J. R. Smith, 1849, p. 105; M. A. Murray, "Egyptian Finger-Counting Rhymes," *Folklore*, vol. 36, no. 2, June 30, 1925, pp. 186–87.

100 *Edwardian nurseries*: "A. R.," *N&Q*, August 15, 1925, p. 122.

101 digitus/daktylos: Ian Whitelaw, *A Measure of All Things: The Story of Man and Measurement*, New York: St. Martin's Press, 2007, pp. 10–12.

101 *Apuleius*: *Apologia*, 89:21–27, for which see Williams and Williams, "Finger
     Numbers in the Greco-Roman World and the Early Middle Ages," p. 596.

101 *Roman system of finger-counting*: *Pace* Menninger, who says the Romans "were
     very poor at computations" (*Number Words and Number Symbols*, p. 36). For
     this section I am indebted to his "Finger Counting," (pp. 201–20), as well as
     to the clear exposition of Edward A. Bechtel, "Finger-Counting among the
     Romans in the Fourth Century," *Classical Philology*, vol. 4, no. 1, January 1909,
     pp. 25–31; Leon J. Richardson, "Digital Reckoning among the Ancients,"
     American Mathematical Monthly, vol. 23, no. 1, January 1916, pp. 7–13; Elisa-
     beth Alföldi-Rosenbaum, "The Finger Calculus in Antiquity and the Middle
     Ages," *Frühmittelalterliche Studien: Jahrbuch des Instituts für Frühmittelalterfor-
     schung der Universität Münster*, vol. 5, 1971, pp. 1–9; Calvin C. Clawson, "How
     Do We Count?" chap. 1 of his *The Mathematical Traveler: Exploring the Grand
     History of Numbers*, New York and London: Plenum Press, 1994, pp. 5–17,
     and Burma P. Williams and Richard S. Williams, "Finger Numbers in the
     Greco-Roman World and the Early Middle Ages," *Isis*, vol. 86, no. 4, De-
     cember 1995, pp. 587–608, who provide an invaluable compendium of "An-
     cient References to Finger Mathematics" (with excellent translations) and an
     equally useful handlist of "Medieval References to Finger Mathematics," that
     is, all the surviving manuscript texts of Bede, with significant variants. See
     also J. A. Picton, "Anglo-Saxon Numerals," *N&Q*, 6th series, vol. 7, June 2,
     1883, p. 433; J. H. Rivett-Carnac, "Numerals," *N&Q*, 9th series, vol. 12, No-
     vember 14, 1903, pp. 387–88; James Walton, "Primitive Counting Systems in
     Use in England," *N&Q*, June 28, 1941, pp. 459–60.

102 *De loquela per gestum digitorum*: See Eva Matthews Sanford, "De Loquela
     Digitorum," *Classical Journal*, vol. 23, no. 8, May 1928, pp. 588–93; Anto-
     nio Quacquarelli, "Al margine dell'actio: la loquela digitorum," *Vetera Chris-
     tianorum*, vol. 7, no. 1, 1970, pp. 199–224; Michael S. Mahoney, "Mathematics,"
     chap. 5 of David C. Lindberg, ed., *Science in the Middle Ages* (The Chicago
     History of Science and Medicine), Chicago: Chicago University Press, 1978,
     pp. 146–50; Francisca del Mar Plaza Picón and José Antonio Gonzáles Marr-
     ero, "'De Computo uel Loquela Digitorum': Beda y el cómputo digital,"
     Faventia: Revista de Filologia clàssica, no. 28, fasc. 1–2, 2006, pp. 115–23.

102 *"1 = the little finger"*: This tally has been adapted from Bechtel's digest, with
     adjustments for clarity.

105 *"10 (a + b) + cd"*: Richardson's old account of the Wallachian "system" is far
     more exhaustive than this, but I have here attempted to account for its prin-
     cipal features as simply as possible. The several larger points of interpretation
     are naturally mine.

107 *knots (as in pre-Columbian America)*: Charles C. Mann, "Unraveling Khipu's
     Secrets," *Science*, vol. 309, no. 5737, August 12, 2005, pp. 1008–9.

109 *Michael Baxandall*: *Painting and Experience in Fifteenth Century Italy: A Primer*

in the Social History of Pictorial Style, Oxford: Oxford University Press (The Clarendon Press), 1972.

109 *the philosopher Favorinus and the jurist Sextus Caecilius Africanus*: Richard A. Bauman, *Crime and Punishment in Ancient Rome*, London: Routledge, 1996, pp. 145–47. See also Ronald T. Ridley, "Appendix 2: *The Twelve Tables*," *History of Rome: A Documented Analysis* (Problemi e ricerche di storia antica, 8), Rome: L'Erma di Bretschneider, 1987, pp. 88–91.

110 yubitsume: A hideous variant of this practice arose from the expectation in seventeenth-century Edo that female prostitutes should demonstrate their loyalty and devotion to certain male clients by spectacularly lopping off one of their own fingers: Lawrence Rogers, "She Loves Me, She Loves Me Not: *Shinju* and *Shikoda Okagami*," *Monumenta Nipponica*, vol. 49, no. 1, 1994, pp. 31–60.

110 *Money*: I have found the most convenient point of access to this vast subject in William N. Goetzmann and K. Geert Rouwenhurst, eds., *The Origins of Value: The Financial Innovations That Created Modern Capital Markets*, Oxford: Oxford University Press, 2005.

111 *Paper money*: Richard van Glahn, "The Origins of Paper Money in China," ibid., pp. 65–89.

111 instrumentum ex causa cambii: Peter Spufford, Wendy Wilkinson, and Sarah Tolley, *A Handbook of Medieval Exchange* (Royal Historical Society Guides and Handbooks, 13), London: Royal Historical Society, 1986, pp. xxx–xxxi.

111 *David Venables*: POB, t16960708–27.

112 *Sarah Willis and Ann Sydney*: POB, t17980912–18.

112 *Thomas and Matilda Miller*: POB, t18060917–15.

113 *many byways of superstition*: See Frank Baker, "Anthropological Notes on the Human Hand," *American Anthropologist*, vol. 1, no. 1, January 1888, pp. 55–59.

6. Gloves

117 *Hull*: King Charles IV of Spain (1748–1819), *N&Q*, 1st series, vol. 5, no. 118, January 31, 1852, p. 102, citing William Hull, Jr., *The History of the Glove Trade, with the customs connected with the glove, to which are annexed some observations on the policy of the trade between England and France, and its operation on the agricultural and manufacturing interests* (London: Effingham Wilson, 1834), who in turn cited Laure Junot, duchesse d'Abrantès, *Mémoires de Madame la Duchesse d'Abrantès, Souvenirs historiques sur Napoléon, la révolution, le directoire, le consulat, l'empire et la restauration*, Paris: Garnier Frères, 1831–34, tome viii, p. 35.

118 Hosier and Glover: A full but brief run is in the Bodleian Library, Oxford.

118 *P. F. Sole*: *The Times*, June 2, 1836, p. 8.

119 *"now fashionable 'bronze-green' silk gloves"*: X. Y. Z., letter to the editor of *The Times*, August 20, 1878, p. 6, and Dent, Allcroft's reply, August 27, p. 8.

119 *duties paid on imported gloves*: See *The Times*, June 26, 1828, p. 7. In fact, for a hundred years, on both sides of the Atlantic, the question of customs duties payable on gloves, glove leather, and glove "fasteners" regularly cropped up. See "Latest Customs Rulings," *NYT*, December 27, 1905, p. 10, where it was reported that foreign metal glove "fasteners" were found not to be assessable as "manufactures of glass" at an astonishingly high rate of 60 percent *ad valorem*, but as "buttons" at 45 percent. See also *NYT*, April 25, 1908, p. 13; "The Duties on Gloves," *NYT*, March 27, 1909, p. 8.

119 *appropriate level of protection*: See "The Dumping of German Gloves," *The Times*, April 18, 1922, p. 12, in which it was reported that a greater degree of protection was sought for the American product, and "British and Foreign Gloves," *The Times*, August 28, 1925, p. 8, in which, writing to the editor, a "glove manufacturer" hotly protested the superiority of the British article over the far cheaper French.

120 *early Christian hand-covering*: The most famous examples in art are the sixth-century mosaics in Ravenna, especially Emperor Justinian and his retinue in S. Vitale, and numerous full-length figures on each side of the nave of the Basilica of S. Apollinare Nuovo, including the three magi, all of whom cover at least one of their hands when offering or carrying holy books, offerings, or the elements of the Eucharist, though intriguingly not Empress Theodora (S. Vitale, with chalice).

120 *Council of Aix*: Isaac Disraeli, "History of Gloves," in *Curiosities of Literature: Consisting of Anecdotes, Characters, Sketches, and Observations, Literary, Critical, and Historical*, London: Printed for J. Murray . . . , 1791, p. 63.

120 *King Magnus Barefoot, King Edward I "Longshanks," and King Henry IV*: Collins, *Love of a Glove*, pp. 31–34.

121 *three countries were needed to make the finest gloves*: Ibid., p. 34.

121 *Mary of Austria*: Ibid., p. 22.

121 *Catherine de Medicis*: Ibid., pp. 18–21.

121 *Queen Elizabeth I*: See also Peter Stallybrass and Ann Rosalind Jones, "Fetishizing the Glove in Renaissance Europe," *Critical Inquiry*, vol. 28, no. 1, Autumn 2001, pp. 114–32, and Aileen Ribeiro, *Fashion and Fiction: Dress in Art and Literature in Stuart England*, New Haven and London: Yale University Press for the Paul Mellon Centre for Studies in British Art, 2005, pp. 50–51; 203 ("perfumed gloves that are lyned," 1605); 66 ("gloves as sweet as damask roses," *The Winter's Tale*, c. 1611, act IV, sc. iii); 67 (re. Paul van Somer, *Elizabeth, Countess of Kellie*, New Haven: Yale Center for British Art, "gauntlet tops embroidered with pearls and sequins on carnation silk"); 94, 96 (re. Daniel Mytens's *King Charles I*, London: National Portrait Gallery, wearing gloves of soft, supple "Cordovan [Spanish] leather"); 134 (re. leather glove with gaily colored silk ribbons, Claydon House, Buckinghamshire: Verney Collection, pl. 136).

122 *Dutch painters:* The following works recently seen in London and The Hague (Rudi Ekkart and Quentin Buvelot, *Dutch Portraits: The Age of Rembrandt and Frans Hals,* translated by Beverly Jackson, London: National Gallery Company, 2007): Frans Hals's *Double Portrait of Isaac Massa and Beatrix van der Laen,* c. 1622 (Amsterdam: Rijksmuseum), no. 15, pp. 106–107, and his *Portrait of Aletta Hanemans,* 1625 (The Hague: Koninklijke Kabinet van Schilderijen, Mauritshuis), no. 17, pp. 110–11, 113 (holding a fancy glove in her left hand); Bartholomeus van der Helst's *Portrait of the Regents of the Voetboogdoelen,* 1656 (Amsterdams Historisch Museum), no. 30, pp. 142–43 (one of whom holds a pair of gloves in his right hand); Thomas de Keyser's *Portrait of Constantijn Huygens and his Clerk,* 1627 (London: National Gallery), no. 34, pp. 150–51 (both of whom wear a single glove on opposite hands); Jan Miense Molenaar's *Portrait of the Painter's Family,* c. 1635 (Amsterdam/Rijswijk: Netherlands Institute for Cultural Heritage, on loan to the Frans Hals Museum), no. 42, pp. 166–67 (in which the artist portrays himself holding the left glove in his right, which is itself gloved); Rembrandt's *Portrait of Andries de Graeff,* 1639 (Kassel: Staatliche Museen, Gemaldegalerie Alte Meister), no. 56, pp. 198–99, and his *Portrait of Jan Six,* 1654 (Amsterdam: Six Collection), no. 57, pp. 200–201; and Johannes Verspronk's *Portrait of Andries Stilte as a Standard-Bearer,* 1640 (Washington, D.C.: National Gallery of Art, Patrons' Permanent Fund), no. 64, pp. 220–21.

122 *Van Dyck:* Susan J. Barnes et al., *Van Dyck: A Complete Catalogue of the Paintings,* New Haven and London: Yale University Press for the Paul Mellon Centre for Studies in British Art, 2004: on gloves in Van Dyck see p. 356, citing D. R. Smith, *Masks of Wedlock: Seventeenth-Century Dutch Marriage Portraiture,* Ann Arbor: University of Michigan Press, 1982, pp. 87–88. The most spectacular examples (among many) are (from the first Antwerp period) *Portrait of a Man Drawing on His Glove* (Dresden: Gemäldegalerie Alte Meister der Staatlichen Kunstsammlungen, no. I.134, pp. 121–22, left hand); (from the Italian period) *Portrait of Man with a Gloved Hand* (private collection, no. II.84, p. 218, left, very loose-fitting); (from the second Antwerp period) *Peeter Stevens* (The Hague: Koninklijke Kabinet van Schilderijen, Mauritshuis, no. III.133, pp. 353 and 355–56, left hand); *Jan de Wael and his Wife Geertruid de Jode* (Munich: Alte Pinakothek, Bayerische Staatsgemäldesammlungen, no. III.140, pp. 360–61, holding both in his right hand); (the English period) *Self-Portrait with Endymion Porter* (Madrid: Prado, no. IV.6, pp. 432–33, wearing the left); *Anne, Lady Russell, Later Countess of Bedford* (Petworth House, Sussex: Lord Egremont, no. IV.22, pp. 444–45, exquisitely dangling the right, from the cuff); *William Villiers, 2nd Viscount Grandison* (Euston Hall, Suffolk: Duke of Grafton, no. IV.108, p. 515, wearing the right); *Sir Thomas Hanmer* (Weston Park, Staffordshire, no. IV.111, p. 518, wearing the left, and holding the other in the same hand); *Henry Rich, Earl of Holland* (Bowhill, Selkirk:

Duke of Buccleuch, no. IV.136, p. 535, wearing both); *Philip Herbert, Earl of Pembroke* (private collection, no. IV.183, p. 571, wearing the right, and holding the other in the same hand); *Charles Stanley, Lord Strange* (Trustees of the Right Honourable Olive, Countess Fitzwilliam's Chattels Settlement and Lady Juliet Tadgell, no. IV.220, p. 601, wearing the right); *Sir Thomas Wharton* (St. Petersburg: State Hermitage Museum, no. IV.241, pp. 615–16, wearing both); but above all the dazzling *Lord John Stuart and Lord Bernard Stuart, Late Earl of Lichfield* (London: National Gallery, no. IV.221, pp. 602–603, in which Lord Bernard wears the left, and dangles the other from the same hand).

122 *Pieter Nason*: Marieke de Winkel, "'Stuft with Nothing but Vanity': The Connotations of Gloves and Fans," in her *Fashion and Fancy: Dress and Meaning in Rembrandt's Paintings*, Amsterdam: Amsterdam University Press, 2006, pp. 85–90.

122 *Velázquez*: See Dawson W. Carr et al., *Velázquez*, London: National Gallery Company, 2006. *The Lady with a Fan* in the Wallace Collection and *Don Adrián Pulido Pareja*, after 1647 (London: National Gallery), fig. 71, p. 96, are rarities, because, as far as I can see and possibly because of Spanish etiquette (see pp. 128–29), among Velázquez's many sitters only King Philip IV (London: National Gallery, probably 1632, no. 24, pp. 172–73; Madrid: Prado, 1634–35, fig. 20, p. 38; Madrid: Prado, c. 1636, no. 31, pp. 194–95; Castres: Musée Goya, on loan from the Louvre, after 1636, fig. 96, p. 194; Florence: Uffizi, c. 1645, fig. 32, p. 59); Prince Balthasar Carlos (Madrid: Prado, 1634–35, no. 25, pp. 176–79; Madrid: Prado, 1635–36, fig. 97, p. 198; Ickworth: The Bristol Collection, c. 1636, no. 32, pp. 198–99; private collection, 1636–39, no. 27, pp. 182–83; Hampton Court Palace: Royal Collection, 1638–39, fig. 68, p. 93); Spínola (in *The Surrender of Breda*, 1634–35, fig. 22, p. 40, who is gauntleted) and the Count-Duke Olivares (Madrid: Prado, c. 1635, fig. 21, p. 39; New York: Metropolitan Museum of Art, c. 1635–36, no. 26, pp. 180–81) are ever portrayed wearing gloves. In all these instances, however, with only one exception—*Philip IV of Spain in Brown and Silver*, no. 24—the royal or noble sitter is either dressed for battle, hunting, or else mounted on horseback. Presumably *Juan de Mateos*, before 1634 (Dresden: Gemäldegalerie Alte Meister der Staatlichen Kunstsammlungen, fig. 99, p. 202), wears gloves in his capacity as master of the hunt.

122 *Rembrandt: Portrait of Maerten Soolmans*, 1634 (private collection, France), in which the sitter clasps in his left hand a glove by the fingers (de Winkel, pp. 63–64).

122 *Rubens*: C. 1638–40 (Vienna: Kunsthistorisches Museum).

125 *Dutch manners in 1700*: Max von Boehn, *Das Beiwerk der Mode: Spitzen, Fächer, Handschuhe Stöcke, Schirme, Schmuck*, Munich: F. Bruckmann, 1928, p. 90, *cit.* de Winkel, n. 134, p. 288.

125 *Sir Brooke Boothby*: London: Tate Britain.

125 *Reynolds: Miss Mary Hickey*, 1770 (New Haven: Yale Center for British Art, soft brown suède); *Miss Crewe*, c. 1775 (private collection, dove gray); *Lady Worsley*, c. 1776 (Harewood House, Leeds: Earl and Countess of Harewood, buff, for riding); *John Manners, Marquess of Granby*, 1763–65 (Sarasota, Fla.: The John and Mabel Ringling Museum of Art, fawn); *Prince George, with Black Servant*, 1786–87 (Arundel Castle: Duke of Norfolk, white kid).

127 *Lawrence*: For example, *Elizabeth Farren*, c. 1790 (New York: Metropolitan Museum of Art, Bequest of Edward S. Harkness, tan with white stitching and pale lining, wearing the left, and dangling the other from the same hand); *Arthur Atherley*, c. 1792 (Los Angeles: Los Angeles County Museum of Art, William Randolph Hearst Collection, fawn, wearing the right, and holding the other in the same hand); *Francis Osborne, 5th Duke of Leeds*, c. 1796 (private collection, white kid, wearing the left only); *Mrs. Joseph May*, c. 1812 (private collection, holding a yellow pair in her right hand); *Tsar Alexander I of Russia*, 1818–19 (Windsor Castle: Royal Collection, white kid, clasped in front); *King George IV*, 1822 (London: Wallace Collection, kid, tossed over the brim of his upturned high hat); *The 2nd Earl of Harewood*, c. 1823 (Harewood House, Leeds: Earl and Countess of Harewood, clasping a pair in his left hand); *King Charles X of France*, 1825 (Royal Collection, white kid, wearing the right, and holding the other in the same hand).

127 *Napoleon*: The emperor owned at least 240 pairs, many of them lined with ermine.

127 *Charles IV*: See note for "Hull" on p. 242.

129 *a sign of discourtesy*: Sebastián de Covarrubias y Orozco, *Tesoro de la lengua castellano o española*, Madrid: por Luis Sánchez, 1611, p. 453, *cit.* S. W. Singer, "Gloves," *N&Q*, 1st series, vol. 2, no. 41, August 10, 1850, p. 165.

129 *Goya*: *Doña Francisca Vicenta Chollet y Caballero*, 1806 (Pasadena: Norton Simon Museum), also *The Bookseller's Wife*, c. 1805 (Washington, D.C.: National Gallery of Art), likewise above-the-elbow white kid, both arms, with tied laces at the cuff.

129 *La Belle Assemblée*: *La Belle Assemblée, or Bell's Court and Fashionable Magazine Addressed Particularly to the Ladies* commenced publication in 1806. This reference is to vol. 5, April 1812, p. 158. Previously (vol. 3, October 1807, p. 171) "rose, green, purple, salmon, and melbourn brown" were declared mandatory.

129 *Delacroix*: Notably *Louis-Auguste Schwiter*, 1826–30 (London: National Gallery, white kid, wearing the left, and with his right hand holding the other with his red-lined hat).

129 *Ingres*: Georges Vigne, *Ingres*, translated by John Goodman, New York: Abbeville Press, 1995. Mademoiselle Rivière and Mlle. Forestier in Ingres's drawing of *The Forestier Family*, both 1806 (Paris: Louvre, fig. 33, p. 55, and fig. 38, p. 63), wear far-above-the-elbow fingerless gloves. *Madame Panckoucke*, 1811 (Paris: Louvre, fig. 57, p. 85), wears a fawn glove on her right hand. *Edme Bo-*

chet, 1811 (Paris: Louvre, fig. 56, p. 84) wears green gloves; *Count Gouriev*, 1821 (St. Petersburg: State Hermitage Museum, fig. 130, p. 156) wears a mustard on his right, and holds the other in the same hand. The Marquis de Pastoret's white kid gloves sit on the table beside him, 1826 (Chicago: Art Institute, fig. 152, p. 183). *Ferdinand-Philippe, duc d'Orléans*, 1842 and 1843 (private collection, and Versailles: Musée National du Château, respectively, figs. 192 and 193, p. 240), wears one white kid glove on his left hand and holds the other in his right. Four fingers of Mme. Moitessier's orange gloves are just visible on the chair behind her, 1851 (Washington, D.C.: National Gallery of Art, fig. 236, p. 279), as are the Princesse de Broglie's crumpled white kid gloves (in the right foreground), 1853 (New York: Metropolitan Museum of Art, fig. 238, p. 281). A drawing, *Isabelle Guille distributing consecrated wafers*, clearly shows that the child is wearing short gloves on both hands, 1856 (Bayonne: Musée Bonnat, fig. 240, p. 283), while Ingres portrays himself wearing his left glove, and holding the other in the same hand, 1859 (Cambridge, Mass.: Fogg Art Museum, Harvard University, fig. 251, p. 296). *Cfr.* Louis-Léopold Boilly, *Madame d'Aucourt de Saint-Just*, c. 1800 (Lille: Musée des Beaux-Arts), who wears a long rust-colored glove on her left hand.

129 *Stubbs*: Judy Egerton, *George Stubbs, Painter: Catalogue Raisonné*, New Haven and London: Yale University Press for the Paul Mellon Centre for British Art, 2007, for example, *James, Earl of Clanbrassil with his Hunter Mowbray*, c. 1765 (private collection), no. 79, pp. 244–45; *Captain Samuel Sharpe Pocklington with his Wife Pleasance and his Sister Frances*, 1769 (Washington, D.C.: National Gallery of Art), no. 98, pp. 272–73; *Assheton Curzon with his Mare Maria*, 1771 (Paris: Louvre), no. 131, pp. 320–21; *A Conversation: Members of the Milbanke and Melbourne Families*, c. 1770 (London: National Gallery), no. 130, pp. 318–19; and *Lady Lade Exercising an Arabian Horse*, 1793 (The Royal Collection), no. 305, pp. 542–43. Evidently jockeys, grooms, factors, and gamekeepers did not normally wear gloves.

129 *Queen Victoria*: "The Queen and the Worcester Glovers.—(From the *Standard*.)," *The Times*, May 25, 1837, p. 4.

131 *petty thieves*: See, for example, the case of George Jenkins, who on May 16, 1833, was tried at the Old Bailey for the theft in Bristol of a large quantity of ribbon and two pairs of gloves (value 3 shillings), convicted of grand larceny, and sentenced to seven years' transportation. Mary O'Brien (September 5, 1833) and John Wills (April 10, 1834) were luckier: Mary O'Brien was found not guilty of stealing six pairs of men's gloves (value 6 shillings) that belonged to her employer, the harp maker Ignace Vanbever. John Wills, the proprietor of a glove shop, was found not guilty of receiving stolen goods, namely four pairs of gloves (value 10 shillings) belonging to Mr. Arnold the manufacturer: all three cases appear in the *POB*. The problem was still grave thirty years later, when Mark Frump and Henry Leech, both glove cutters,

along with several accomplices, were tried in Birmingham for stealing a number of cape and lamb skins (value 10 shillings) from the establishment of Messrs. Causer and Williams the glove manufacturers, then attempting to remove the identifying stamps with a pumice stone. "The Glove Robberies at Worcester," *Birmingham Daily Post*, April 25, 1865, p. 8.

131 *Eliza Grimwood*, "The Murder at Lambeth," *The Times*, July 4, 1838, p. 6.

131 *delightful spasm of antiquarian interest*: The examples in this paragraph are all taken from "The History of Gloves," a section of Isaac Disraeli's *Curiosities of Literature, Consisting of Anecdotes, Characters, Sketches, and Observations, Literary, Critical, and Historical*, London: John Murray, 1791, pp. 63ff., which was constantly reprinted on both sides of the Atlantic throughout the nineteenth century, and liberally plagiarized as in "A Brief History of Gloves: Ancient and Modern," *Saturday Magazine*, April 17, 1841, pp. 151–52; in the chapter on hosiery in *The Useful Arts Employed in the Production of Clothing*, 2nd ed., London: John W. Parker, 1851, p. 144; "Gloves: Ancient and Modern," *Pall Mall Gazette*, vol. 48, no. 7418, December 26, 1888, pp. 5–6; all the way down to C. Cody Collins in his impressionistic but otherwise useful *Love of a Glove*, New York: Fairchild Publishing Company, 1945, especially pp. 29–30. Disraeli appears to be enjoying a new and unacknowledged lease on life in the article on the history of gloves at wikipedia.com, while he himself borrowed extensively from "the papers of an ingenious antiquary," in *The Present State of the Republic of Letters*, vol. 10, 1728 or 1729, p. 289. The specific references are to Ruth 4:7; Xenophon, *Cyropaedia*, 8:3:17; the glutton is mentioned in the *Deipnosophistae* of Athenaeus, 10; Pliny, *Letters* 4:27:5 (to Baebius Macer); Varro, *De Re Rustica*, 2:55. See also Herodotus, 6:72:1, where Leotychides is bribed with a gauntlet full of silver. The early literature of the history of gloves is broad and fascinating, and includes Vallet d'Artois, *Manuel du fabricant de gants*, 2nd ed., Paris: Roret, 1835; Robert Chambers's *Book of Days, a Miscellany of Popular Antiquities*, London and Edinburgh: W. & R. Chambers 1862, vol. 1, p. 31; S. William Beck, *Gloves: Their Annals and Associations: A Chapter of Trade and Social History*, London: Hamilton, Adams & Co., 1883; Auguste Racinet's *Le Costume historique*, 6 vols., Paris: Firmin-Didot, 1888; Léon Côte's *L'Industrie gantière et l'ouvrier gantier à Grenoble*, with a preface by Jean Jaurès, Paris: G. Bellais, 1903; W. B. Redfern, *Royal and Historic Gloves and Shoes*, London: Methuen, 1904; and Joseph Braun, S.J., *Die liturgische Gewandung im Occident und Orient: Nach Ursprung und Entwicklung, Verwendung und Symbolik*, Freiburg im Breisgau: Herder, 1907, pp. 359–82; Josef Jettmar, *Die Lederhandschuhfabrikation: die Geschichte, die Produktions- und Absatzverhältnisse des Lederhandschuhes in den einzelnen Staaten, seine Rohmaterialien und Herstellung*, Leipzig: Voigt, 1915; George Cecil, "The History of the Glove," *Connoisseur*, vol. 42, 1915, pp. 3–13; and numerous other references provided by contributors to *N&Q*, vol. 149, no. 5, September 5, 1925, p. 177; no. 19, September 19, 1925, p. 214; and no. 20, September 26, 1925, p. 230.

133 chirothocae *and* manicae *or* digitalia: See P. G. W. Glare, ed., *Oxford Latin Dictionary*, Oxford: Oxford University Press, 1983, p. 1073.

133 *Queen Mary*: Calendar of State Papers Foreign—Mary. The gift was sent by Peter Vannes, Queen Mary's ambassador to Venice, to her minister, his colleague Sir William Petre. Gloves were perfumed with musk, ambergris, and other rare perfumes. See Dan[iel]. Hanbury, "Frangipani," *N&Q*, 2nd series, vol. 8, December 24, 1859, pp. 509–11; Septimus Piesse, "Scenting of Books," ibid., 3rd series, vol. 8, September 2, 1865, p. 199 (erroneously claiming that the Earl of Oxford was the first man to bring perfumed gloves to England— for Queen Elizabeth); and his "Ambergris," ibid., 4th series, vol. 1, April 4, 1868, p. 327, noting that Parisian glovers had functioned also as perfumers since the twelfth century at the latest. Georgiana Hill thought perfumed gloves were a "decidedly French" and not a Spanish fashion in the Elizabethan period: "Mundus Muliebris," ibid., 5th series, vol. 1, March 12, 1892, p. 204. Collins (*Love of a Glove*, p. 22) believed that Marguerite of Valois popularized the perfuming of gloves with musk, ambergris, and civet. Nineteenth-century "Limerick gloves" were apparently perfumed with rose petals: Harriet D. Jump, *Routledge Anthology of Nineteenth Century Short Stories by Women*, Florence, Kentucky: Routledge, 1998, p. 33.

133 *King Charles I*: Calendar of State Papers Domestic—Charles I, vol. 279, p. 381. These gloves "were of four sorts:—The first sort were those given to 'the Bishops that consecrate.' If we rightly understand the meaning of some figures in the margin they were compounded for by a payment of 22*s*. to each Bishop. The second sort were to the Doctors and Archdeacon of Canterbury, and the steward, treasurer, and comptroller of the Archbishop's house; the composition of these was 14*s*. The third sort consisted of 12 other members of the Archbishop's household whose composition money was 10*s*. The fourth consisted of 21 servants of inferior order, each of whom received 6*s*."

133 *"challenges of subjective belief, or evidences of objective truth"*: William Bell, "Gloves," *N&Q*, 3rd series, July 12, 1862, pp. 31–32.

134 *white gloves had been presented to a magistrate*: This was still practiced in English courts of law as recently as 1938 ("Two Pairs of White Gloves for the Judge," *The Times*, January 29, p. 7). The custom does not seem to have been known to Beverley Southgate, whose recent article about history and ethics takes as its prompt a reference to it by Lord Acton, who accused the historian Mandell Creighton of wishing to "pass through scenes of raging controversy and passion with a serene curiosity, a suspended judgment, a divided jury, and a pair of white gloves," in other words, of not taking a moral stance in his writing ("'A Pair of White Gloves': Historians and Ethics," *Rethinking History*, vol. 10, no. 1, March 2006, pp. 49–50). Southgate assumes that Acton's reference to white gloves was merely a vague evocation of effete detachment by association with "fashion accessories," and not a specific allusion to the

old ceremonial acknowledgment that there was before the court no pressing matter upon which to render judgment. See also William J. Thoms, "White Gloves at a Maiden Assize," *N&Q*, 1st series, vol. 1, no. 5, December 1, 1849, and the ensuing discussion by M. W., both pp. 72–73; also C. H. Cooper, "Gloves," ibid., 1st series, vol. 3, no. 83, 1851, p. 424; and A. S. J., "Gloves given on Reversal of Outlawry," ibid., 2nd series, vol. 4, no. 79, July 4, 1857, p. 5; and more recently "White Gloves for the Magistrate," *The Times*, June 22, 1914, p. 3 (noting a ceremony that the chief clerk at Guildhall in London had occasion to perform only four times in twenty years). See also Cosmo Innes, *Lectures on Scotch Legal Antiquities*, Edinburgh: Edmonston and Douglas, 1872, pp. 65–66, and Sir James Norton-Kyshe, *The Law and Customs Relating to Gloves*, London: Stevens and Haynes, 1901, *passim*.

134 *Knowles*: The advertisement appeared on Friday, April 17, 1789, p. 2; the "THANKSGIVING DAY" was observed the following Thursday, April 23.

134 *Lafayette*: Thursday, December 30, at Mr. Talbott's Hotel. A pair of "Lafayette" gloves was exhibited most recently at the New-York Historical Society's commemorative exhibition, *French Founding Father: Lafayette's Return to Washington's America*, November 16, 2007–August 10, 2008.

135 *ceremonial gauntlets*: "Gauntlets of Ceremony; Lord Mayor's Visit to Canada; City Companies' Gift," *The Times*, August 8, 1936, p. 7.

135 *duels*: "Four Duels in France," p. 9: the other three were knock-on affairs arising from the Comte de Lubersac's bad temper, and subsidiary insults exchanged between the various seconds. For duels in colonial Australia (principally the Port Phillip District of New South Wales), see Paul Huège de Serville's masterpiece, *Port Phillip Gentlemen and Good Society in Melbourne before the Gold Rushes*, Melbourne: Oxford University Press, 1980, pp. 106–24, 214–16. Judge Redmond Barry wore gloves with his "bell topper," white vest, and swallow-tail coat, when in the winter of 1841 he fought a duel at Sandhurst with the irascible squatter and clubman Peter Snodgrass (pp. 110, 214).

135 *glove-wearing in church . . .*: See F. C. H. in *N&Q*, 2nd series, vol. 5, no. 109, January 30, 1858, pp. 98–99, and J. S. B., ibid., 2nd series, vol. 5, no. 114, March 6, 1858, p. 190; also R. W. Munro, "Preaching in Gloves," ibid., vol. 198, no. 8, August 1953, p. 361.

135 *. . . and at funerals*: Also C., "Notes on Manners, Costume, etc." *N&Q*, 1st series, vol. 10, no. 253, 1854, p. 178 (mourning); A. L. Humphreys, ibid., 7th series, vol. 8, October 12, 1880, p. 293 (documenting the use of gloves, suspended garland-like, as simple memorials to dead children); Alfred Wallis, "Mittens or Gloves as Funeral Decorations," ibid., 7th series, vol. 8, October 12, 1889, pp. 292–93 (i.e., of white paper carried at the funerals of young unmarried women, also the gift of black or, in the case of virgins, white gloves to all present at a funeral); Jonathan Bouchier, "Mittens or Gloves as

Funeral Decorations," ibid., 7th series, vol. 9, January 18, 1890, pp. 52–53 (citing Scott's *Rokeby* [1813], in which Bertram Risingham hangs his steel gauntlet over an altar, not in connection with funerary rites, but as a sacred challenge to whoever was prepared to take it down). I am grateful to Steven C. Bullock, Associate Professor of United States History at the Worcester Polytechnic Institute, Worcester, Mass., for allowing me to read a draft of his essay "A Handsome Mark of Respect: Funeral Glove-Giving in Early New England" (forthcoming).

135 *white gloves* "à la Chopin": Adam Zamoyski, *Chopin*, New York: Doubleday and Co., 1980, p. 113, *cit.* Benita Eisler, *Chopin's Funeral*, Westminster, Md.: Knopf Publishing Group, 2004, pp. 47–48. This was reported by Chopin's friend Antoni Orlowski, who further added that Chopin said "[my] carriage and white gloves alone cost more than I can earn."

136 *Anglican bishop*: The Right Reverend John C. Vockler, Bishop of Polynesia (1962–68). I am grateful to the Right Reverend Andrew St. John, D.D., for this amusing recollection. See also Joseph Braun, "Episcopal Gloves," *The Catholic Encyclopedia*, New York: Robert Appleton Company, 1909, vol. 6, pp. 589–90.

136 *French army*: November 3, p. 21, citing the *Pall Mall Gazette*.

136 *correct form at Court or in church*: See John R. Magrath, "Gloves: Survivals of Old Customs," *N&Q*, 12th series, vol. 2, October 28, 1918, p. 356. The discussion about not wearing gloves in the presence of royalty had been going on since 1850 at the latest: See F. E., "Why are Gloves not worn before Royalty?" ibid., 1st series, vol. 1, no. 23, 1850, p. 366; W. Dn., ibid., 1st series, vol. 2, no. 58, December 7, 1850, p. 467; Philip S. King, ibid., 1st series, vol. 5, no. 118, January 31, 1852, p. 102; and C., ibid., 1st series, vol. 5, no. 120, February 14, 1852, p. 157. Notwithstanding the opinion frequently expressed that women should not wear gloves in the presence of royalty, the evidence of later Court photographers and nearly contemporary engravings is unequivocal: women did wear them when presented at formal "courts" of the Edwardian period, especially debutantes. See Nigel Arch and Joanna Marschner, *Splendour at Court: Dressing for Royal Occasions since 1700*, London: Unwin Hyman, 1987, p. 105.

137 *working women*: See "A Matter of Gloves," *NYT*, February 1, 1903, p. SM13.

137 *Rhode Island*: "Gloves in Summer," ibid., July 23, 1907, p. 6.

137 *Queen Alexandra*: "The Inartistic White Glove," ibid., July 26, 1908, p. X7.

137 *gloves at their weddings*: "Women Discard Gloves," ibid., May 16, 1909, p. C2.

138 *increasingly flamboyant range of styles*: The references are given here in date order: (1916) "Summer Fashion Hints," *NYT*, July 2, p. X2; (1921) Sara Marshall Cook in the *Washington Post*, January 23, p. 47; (1922) Mary Brush Williams, "The Last Word in Paris Fashions," *Chicago Daily Tribune*, November 19, p. C1; (1923) Mary O'Connor Newell, "Fashion Hints," *Washington Post*, May 23, p. 10; (1924) "London Fashions: Gloves and Shoes," *The Times*,

April 30, p. 17; (1925) "Gloves That Are Smart: Conventional Hand Coverings of Recent Years Have Quite Given Way to Gay and Attractive New Modes," *NYT*, February 1, p. 10.

139 *glove lengths apparently crept ever upward*: (1929) "Gloves Achieve Importance among Autumn Accessories: They Are Being Promoted for Evening Wear as Well as for Sports and Street," *Washington Post*, July 7, p. S7; Honore Booth, "Modes of the Moment," *Los Angeles Times*, December 2, p. A8; Vyella Poe Wilson, *Washington Post*, December 8, 1929, p. S9; (1930) "London Fashions: Gloves and Hats," *The Times*, March 19, p. 17; (1932) "Gloves Conform to Dress Mode," *NYT*, August 21, 1932, p. 6; (1933) "London Fashions: Gloves and Shoes," *The Times*, May 10, p. 17; (1934) "Round the Shops ... Gloves and Shoes," ibid., October 25, p. 9; (1936) Marie Mossoba, "Old Romance of the Glove: The Gay Hues of Today Recall the Bright Hand-Coverings Worn in a Glamorous Past," *NYT*, May 10, p. SM15.

140 *violet-blue gloves with notes of black or ... thunder-gray* (1939): "The Fascination of Gloves: Colours for Every Mood," *The Times*, January 20, p. 17; Prince Jean-Louis de Faucigny-Lucinge, *Legendary Parties*, New York: The Vendôme Press, 1987, pp. 39–42; (1940) Kathleen Cannell, "Gloves Important in New Spring Styles," *NYT*, February 11, p. 56, and her "Paris to Show Styles in Holland," ibid., April 7, p. 55 (in both instances reporting from Paris).

140 *harbingers of prosperity*: (1946) "Fashion Points to Gloves as Costume Complements," *NYT Studio*, January 8, p. 26; (1949) "Fashion Limelight Swings to Gloves," ibid., April 18, p. 17; "Rich Accessories Offered in Show," ibid., November 4, p. 30; "Unusual Fabrics Diversify Gloves," ibid., November 29, p. 34; (1950) *Vogue*, March 15, n.p. [advertisement].

141 *gray-and-yellow*: (1954) *Vogue*, September 1, p. 204; (1956) "On Hand for Spring: Lean Look, Discreet Detail," *NYT*, February 6, p. 16; (1957) "Colored Glove Elbowing Way into High Fashion," *NYT*, October 16, p. 39.

141 *sultry tobacco-smoking*: Jim Heimann, ed., *50s All-American Ads*, with an introduction by Jim Heimann, Cologne, London, etc.: Taschen, 2001: Marlene Dietrich, 1950, p. 86; Ascot cigarette lighters, handled by women wearing long pink, green, and black gloves, p. 94; Lucille Ball (in white gloves) for Philip Morris, "You'll be glad tomorrow ... you smoked Philip Morris today," p. 95.

142 *crackers*: Ritz, 1950, ibid., p. 633; *automobiles*: Cadillac 1954, p. 206; 1956, pp. 238, 258, and 1958, pp. 272–73, 290; Pontiac 1958, pp. 232–33; Lincoln 1959, p. 293; Imperial LeBaron Silvercrest 1959, pp. 310–11; Oldsmobile 1959, pp. 312–13; *beer*: "'My beer is Rheingold—the *Dry* beer!' says Madelyn Darrow, Miss Rheingold 1958," p. 52; Schlitz, "World's largest selling beer, the beer that made Milwaukee famous," 1956, p. 53; *soft furnishings*: Leather industries of America, 1950, p. 797.

142 *Immensely long, twenty-button glacé kid or skinny green gloves*: (1958) Evelyn

Livingstone, "Color in Fall Accessories," *Chicago Daily Tribune*, July 17, p. C5; "French Style Expert Calls Gloves Principal Accessory in Wardrobe," *NYT*, October 27, p. 35 (Mme. De Nervo); "Caught Red Handed!" [Kayser advertisement] in *Vogue*, September 1; "Dawnelle" [advertisement], *Vogue*, October 15.

142 *Kislav*: (1961) Marylin Bender, "French Keep Glove Secret Under Guard," *NYT*, August 21, p. 17; (1964) Bernardine Morris, "Gloves Aim 'to Amuse,' Not Match," *NYT*, March 19, p. 36 ("Elayne"). The story may not be over: An article by R. Coggins in *Good Housekeeping*, vol. 213, no. 4, October 1991, p. 54, announced "The Return of the Glove," and gloves were quite prominent in the North American fall season of 2007: Lynn Yaeger, "A Show of Hands," *Vogue*, September, p. 554. A month earlier, the late Brooke Astor was the subject of a special photographic tribute in the Sunday Style section of the *NYT* (Bill Cunningham, "To the Nines," August 19, 2007, p. 4), in which it was noted that Mrs. Astor's "signature" was a pair of white kid gloves, freshly laundered for her in Paris.

143 *A. T. Gallico*: This gathering of advice from the heavily sponsored A. T. Gallico in the *Chicago Daily Tribune* serves to demonstrate the extraordinary persistence of glove fashions for men in the Roaring Twenties: "Men's Fashions," *Chicago Daily Tribune*, November 23, 1923, p. 22 (chamoisette, and chamoisette of double weight, called "duplex"); "Men's Fashions: To Be Well-Gloved," ibid., April 2, 1924, p. 22 (tan cape, gray mocha, natural or drab buckskin, white dress, and gray suede gloves); "Men's Fashions: Gloves for Sport," ibid., April 8, 1924, p. 27 ("golf gloves are now sold in a color exactly the shade of clay dust … Gloves for polo have tan cape palms with white buckskin backs"); "Men's Fashions: Red Lined Gloves," ibid., April 29, 1924, p. 23 (buckskin, lined with red silk: "It is more an affair for a stroll down some quiet lane or avenue that needs cheering up. Doubtless the wearer pauses every block or two, peeks under the flap of his glove, is refreshed by the glowing scarlet, and marches on, feeling better and happier"); "Men's Fashions: White Gloves for Night Driving," ibid., May 26, 1924, p. 23 ("the more white gloves the motorist buys and wears, the longer he will live to buy more white gloves"); "Men's Fashions: For Night Motorists," ibid., October 9, 1924, p. 23 (offering an alternative solution to the problem of wearing white gloves while driving at night: "an ordinary pair of gloves with a single red reflector affixed to the back of the left hand, for easily visible manual indication"); "Men's Fashions: Your Glove Requirements," ibid., January 8, 1925, p. 22 (recommending for the winter season tan cape or buck gloves of gray, tan, fawn, or white … white kid or white cape or suede, or gray suede. "But if the evening affair is quite ceremonious, such as ushering or best manning at a wedding, the white kid are necessary"); "Men's Fashions: Always the Glove," ibid., July 27, 1925, p. 23 (chamois or doeskin gloves in white or extremely

light natural chamois color, with black stitching in wide stitches, paired with light colored spats); "Men's Fashions," ibid., February 10, 1925, p. 23 ("Reddish tan is coming greatly into favor, while brown is dying out. The mocha gloves are most popular in lighter shades of gray. Natural buckskin gloves of pearly tint are among the most popular handwear, as well as buckskin gloves in shades such as camel, buff, and fawn"); "Men's Fashions: Attention to Gloves," ibid., October 14, 1925, p. 26 ("The average man . . . [knows] . . . enough not to wear white kid gloves with a tweed topcoat"); "Men's Fashions: Glove Ways and Means," ibid., November 18, 1925, p. 23 ("If you have large hands and do not wish to call attention to the fact, avoid wearing light colored gloves for the same reason that you avoid light colored spats or shoes if you are sensitive about big feet"); and "Men's Fashions: Chamois Glove Is Smart," ibid., December 2, 1925, p. 25 ("Of course, there are gloves and gloves . . . the chamois glove with black stitching, in either the pull-on or button variety . . . is a smart-looking glove for street wear, but being rather a conspicuous glove should not be worn by anyone who is anxious to conceal the size of his hands").

143   *denim*: For this shrewd observation I am indebted to my colleague Patricia E. Kane; personal communication with the author.

143   *worlds of total unreality*: "Wardrobe of Gloves Suggested," *NYT*, November 15, 1962, p. 62.

146   *Degas, Whistler, and Sargent*: Degas: Gloves are almost certainly worn by both gentlemen in the *Place de la Concorde*, 1875 (St. Petersburg: State Hermitage Museum), and by Alexis Rouart in *Henri Rouart and His Son Alexis*, 1895–98 (Munich: Neue Pinakothek), who, standing, is either putting them on or taking them off. See also *Singer with a Glove*, c. 1878 (Cambridge, Mass.: Fogg Art Museum, Wertheim Collection, Harvard University), and most of the millinery scenes, for example, *The Millinery Shop*, c. 1884–90 (Chicago: Art Institute of Chicago, Mr. and Mrs. Lewis Larned Coburn Memorial Collection). Much of the power of *L'Absinthe*, 1875–76 (Paris: Musée d'Orsay) is surely due to the clever concealment of the hands, drooping hopelessly in the drinker's lap, beneath the table. Her male companion is not wearing gloves. Whistler: *Arrangement in Black and Gold: Comte Robert de Montesquiou-Fezensac*, for which see Edgar Munham, *Whistler and Montesquiou: The Butterfly and the Bat*, New York and Paris: Frick Collection and Flammarion, 1995, *passim*. Sargent: for example, *Mrs. Joseph Chamberlain*, 1902 (Washington, D.C.: National Gallery of Art), long white kid, and *Portrait of Ena Wertheimer: A Vele Gonfie*, 1905 (London: Tate Britain, bequeathed by Robert Mathias), long, snugly fitting black glacé, on the right hand, a tour-de-force of painterly brilliance.

146   *Mme. Cézanne*: *Madame Cézanne in the Conservatory*, 1891 (New York: Metropolitan Museum of Art, Bequest of Stephen C. Clark), is a rare exception. Mme. Cézanne here wears mid-arm-length black semitransparent, fingerless

gloves, possibly of lace, which were old-fashioned: as an old lady, Marceline Desbordes-Valmore wore a similar pair in 1854 when she was the subject of the earliest documented photograph by Nadar. See Maria Morris Hambourg et al., *Nadar*, New York: Metropolitan Museum of Art, 1995, pl. 24, and p. 229.

146 *Dr. Gachet*: Dr. *Gachet*, by Vincent van Gogh, in two versions, both June 1890 (private collection and Paris: Musée d'Orsay).

146 *Picasso's women*: See William Rubin, ed., *Picasso and Portraiture: Representation and Transformation*, New York: The Museum of Modern Art, 1996: *Portrait of Gertrude Stein*, 1906 (New York: Metropolitan Museum of Art, Bequest of Gertrude Stein), p. 267; *Dora Maar Seated*, 1937 (Paris: Musée Picasso; Zervos VIII, 331), p. 391. For the same year's *Guernica* see pp. 22 and 26 above.

146 *Edward Hopper*: For example, *Automat*, 1927 (Des Moines, Iowa: Des Moines Art Center).

146 *Gilbert and George*: Carter Ratcliff and Robert Rosenblum, *Gilbert and George: The Singing Sculpture*, New York: Anthony McCall, 1993, *passim*.

146 *Boldini's* Montesquiou: Paris: Musée d'Orsay.

7. Nail Polish

149 *champagne bottles*: Jim Heimann, ed., *50s All-American Ads*, with an introduction by Jim Heimann, Cologne, London, etc.: Taschen, 2001: "Moët," 1952, p. 63; *carnations*: Lustre-Creme Shampoo, as used by Elizabeth Taylor (with pink nails and prominent wedding band no. 3, viz. Mike Todd), 1957, p. 385; *beach balls*: Coronet magazine, n.d., p. 35; "Avon," 1957, p. 366; *chlorophyll toothpaste*: by Colgate, 1952, p. 367; "Soft Weve," 1953, p. 369; "Lady Sunbeam," ibid., 1957, p. 372; *big-range cooking*, ibid.: General Electric Range, 1956, pp. 404–405; *office machines*: Western Electric telephone handsets, featuring "past" (no nail polish), present (pink), and an oddly shaped "future?" (powder blue), p. 744; Gilbert office papers, 1955, p. 748; Royal Portable Typewriters, 1955, p. 749; National adding machines, n.d., p. 758; *domestic appliances*: Admiral refrigerators, 1956, p. 392; Sunbeam ironmaster, 1957, p. 444; "sofas" by Kroehler, 1955, "metallic nylon fabrics in exciting new colors!" p. 790; *"pert and perky" foundation garments and swimming suits*: Perma-lift, 1957, p. 545; Catalina, 1954, pp. 541, 543; *nylons*: bur-mil Cameo stockings, "The hue is the cry," 1958, p. 607; *insecticides*: Black Flag bug killer, 1950, p. 466; *Coca-Cola*, 1952, p. 670; *Pepsi*, 1953 and 1959, p. 680; *television sets*: Philco, 1957, p. 437; *candy, canned and frozen food*: Brach's chocolates, 1950, p. 647; Chun King Chow Mein and Chop Suey, 1953, p. 641; *Cheez Whiz*, 1956, a particularly revolting form of instant macaroni cheese, pp. 644–45; PictSweet frozen fresh sliced strawberries, 1957, p. 667; *patio furniture*: Owens Corning fiberglass, 1956, pp. 794–95.

150 *burlesque*: The cover of *Cabaret Quarterly*, vol. 6, n.d., and ibid., p. 33; "hospital and operating theater," A.L. Stainless steel, 1955, pp. 698–99.

151 *But what exactly is it?*: In this section I am indebted to the following: Jay M. Barnett and Richard K. Scher, "Nail Cosmetics," *International Journal of Dermatology*, vol. 31, no 10, October 1992, pp. 675–81; Maurice J. Dahdah and Richard K. Scher, "Nail Diseases Related to Nail Cosmetics," *Dermatologic Clinics*, vol. 24, 2006, pp. 233–39; Steven Greenhouse, "Studies Highlight Hazards of Manicurists' Chemicals," *NYT*, August 19, 2007, p. A26; Warren R. Heymann, "Nail Cosmetics: Potential Hazards," *Journal of the American Academy of Dermatology*, vol. 57, 2007, pp. 1069–70; and Meena Moossavi and Richard K. Scher, "Nail Care Products," *Clinics in Dermatology*, vol. 19, 2001, pp. 445–48. The industry has a powerful voice, for example that of Francis Busch of ProStrong, Inc.: "Multifunctional Nail Care Products," in Randy Schueller, *Multifunctional Cosmetics*, New York: Marcel Dekker, 2002, pp. 99–114. Other scientists such as Phoebe Rich, "Nail Cosmetics," *Dermatologic Clinics*, vol. 24, 2006, pp. 393–99, are far more sanguine as to the risks than the majority: "Nail cosmetics," she writes, "are not inherently dangerous." See also Natasha Singer, "Nail Polish Makers Yield on Disputed Chemical," *NYT*, September 7, 2006, p. 3.

154 *Victorian fashion literature*: Blanche Soyer, baronne Staffe, *Lady's Dressing Room*, translated . . . by Lady Colin Campbell, London: Cassell and Company, 1892.

154 *French ladies of the ancien régime*: Ibid., pp. 183–84.

155 Le Misanthrope: Charles A. Eggert, ed., *Molière's Le Misanthrope*, Boston: D. C. Heath and Co., 1902, p. 123. The comment continues: "E. Fournier quotes from a 'receuil,' published in 1661: 'la belle mode qui courut parmi nos godelureaux de laisser croître l'ongle du petit doigt.' Scarron (1610–60) mentions it in connection with one of his characters (*Nouvelles tragic-comiques*, p. 4, 1665)." The original passage, in its incomparably elegant couplets, runs: *"Mais au moins, dites-moi, madame, par quel sort / votre Clitandre a l'heur de vous plaire si fort? / Sur quell fonds de mérite et de vertu sublime / Appuyez-vous en lui l'honneur de votre estime? / Est-ce que par l'ongle long qu'il porte au petit doigt / Qu'il s'est acquis chez vous l'estime où l'on le voit?"* It was also noticed that by shifting the adjective *long* from its normal position before the noun, Molière laid particular emphasis upon the elongated nail of Clitandre's little finger. See also G. Masson and "Alpha," "The Nail of the Little Finger Left to Grow (6th S. vii. 50)," *N&Q*, 6th series, vol. 7, April 21, 1883, pp. 316–17.

155 *fat hands*: *Lady's Dressing Room*, p. 194.

155 Pall Mall Gazette: "A Believer in Palmistry," "Tell-Tale Fingers," *The Pall Mall Gazette*, March 4, 1886, p. 4.

157 *seventeenth-century Japan*: Kumagusu Minakata, "Finger-Metal," *N&Q*, March 24, 1928, p. 209: "In Burton's 'Anatomy of Melancholy,' mem. 2, subs. 2, we

read: 'A little soft hand, pretty little mouth, small, fine, long fingers, *Gratiae quae digitis*—'tis that which Apollo did admire in Daphne—*laudat digitosque manusque* [Ovid, *Metamorphoses*].' That similarly the Japanese of the seventeenth century made much of such fingers is obvious in Saikwaku's 'Ichidai Otoko,' 1682, tome iii, ch. 2, where it is said 'In Kyoto beautiful girls are reared from infancy with the face repeatedly steamed, and while in bed, putting "finger-metal" on each finger and socks on the feet.' This 'finger-metal' (*yubigane*) seems to have been a device for shaping the fingers, small, fine, and slender, by peripheral compression, but nowadays nowhere in the empire can it be found."

157 *"Beautiful nails are looked upon as a precious gift"*: *Lady's Dressing Room*, pp. 205–206.

157 *The art of the* manicure: See, for example, Anon., "The 'Manicure,'" *Daily Evening Bulletin* (San Francisco), May 20, 1876, n.p., col. D.; Anon., "The Mysteries of Beauty: How to Become Beautiful—The Secret of the Dermatologist and the Manicure—A Lady's [anonymous] Visit to the Sanctum of Prof. Cameron [in Parlor no. 10, Hurst's Hotel]," *St. Louis Globe-Democrat*, April 3, 1881, p. 286; Anon., "The Manicure: A Practical Demonstration of the Art of Shaping and Beautifying the Finger Nails," *St. Louis Globe-Democrat*, January 12, 1884, p. 4; Anon., "The Manicure for Gentlemen," *Atchison Daily Champion*, June 26, 1888, p. 6 (underlining the importance of shininess); Anon., "Princess of Wales's Manicure," *Bismarck Daily Tribune*, December 22, 1889, p. 4 ("a quiet, unobtrusive little French woman"); Anon., "Talks with a Manicure: Cold Weather Advice for the Hands, Lips, Nails, and Hair," *Milwaukee Journal*, December 19, 1894, p. 4.

158 *applied it liberally to their cheeks*: Anon., "It Had to Wear Off: Young Ladies Who Tried Manicure Powder on Their Cheeks," *Yenowine's Illustrated News*, March 5, 1893, p. 2.

158 Milwaukee Sentinel: Anon., "The Thumb and Toe: How the Manicure Goes to Work to Beautify Them," March 19, 1883, p. 6.

158 *Feast of St. Philibert*: OED, *cfr.* the German variant *Lamberts-nuss*. See also Walter W. Skeat, "Filbert (9th S. ix. 125)," *N&Q*, 9th series, vol. 9, March 1, 1902, p. 177.

159 *"The Lady Rohesia"*: *The Ingoldsby Legends; or, Mirth and Marvels*, Philadelphia: Willis P. Hazard, 1856, vol. 1, p. 264.

159 Framley Parsonage: vol. 1, chap. 1, p. 7.

159 *Mrs. Craik*: Dinah Maria Craik (1826–87), "The Woman's Kingdom: A Love Story," *Good Words*, vol. 9, November 1, 1868, p. 665 (coming at the end of chap. 28).

159 *"His Princess"*: John Strange Winter, "His Princess," in *Cavalry Life, or Sketches and Stories in Barracks and Out*, London: Chatto and Windus, 1884, p. 182.

160 *filbert nails denoted high birth*: Henry Syer Cuming, "Finger-Nail Lore," *Journal of the British Archaeological Association*, vol. 40, 1884, pp. 382–83.

160 *British nurse*: Julia Prinsep Stephen, *Notes from Sick Rooms*, London: Smith, Elder and Co., 1883, p. 17.

160 *the paragon of the mature woman*: *Every Saturday: A Journal of Choice Reading*, vol. 7, February 6, 1869, p. 180.

161 *dedicated spiritualist and table-rapper*: Elliott O'Donnell, *Byways of Ghost Land*, London: William Rider and Son, 1911, pp. 162–63.

161 *symmetry, and neatness as well*: See also J. Waring-Curran, "In-Growth of the Toe-Nail," *The Retrospect of Practical Medicine and Surgery*, part 62, January 1871, p. 131.

161 *"pulmonary consumption"*: E. Harris Ruddock, "Phthisis Pulmonalis (*Phthisis Pulmonalis*) Pulmonary Consumption," *The Homeopathic Vade Mecum of Modern Medicine and Surgery*, London: Jarrold and Sons, 12, Paternoster Row, 1871, p. 242.

161 *Dr. James Startin*: "A Course of Lectures on Diseases of the Skin," *The Medical Times*, no. 328, January 10, 1846, p. 291.

162 Judy, or, The London Serio-Comic Journal: Vol. 33, December 26, 1883, p. 301.

162 *Dr. Charles Hilton Fagge*: Author, with Philip Henry Pye-Smith, of "Affections of the Nails," *A Text-Book of Medicine*, London: J. & A. Churchill, 1902, vol. 2, p. 947.

162 *"The Management of the Finger-Nails"*: [Lewis] "Durlacher," *Chambers's Edinburgh Journal*, vol. 90, September 1845, p. 192, *cfr.* "The Toilette and Ladies' Guide," *Bow Bells*, vol. 4, no. 98, June 1866, p. 477—copied verbatim from Dr. Durlacher. This popular article seems to have been a condensation of Lewis Durlacher's *Treatise on Corns, Bunions, the Diseases of Nails and the General Management of the Feet*, London: Simpkin, Marshall, and Co., 1845.

163 *"Every woman likes pink nails"*: Edna K. Forbes, "Beauty Chats: Manicure Helps," *Atlanta Constitution*, January 29, 1925, p. 16. See also Anon., "Short Sleeves Require Lovely Arms and Hands: Nails Are Part of the Charming Ensemble; Rose, Opalescent and Jewel Tints in Polish," *Washington Post*, June 1, 1930, p S8.

165 *"Will you have two coatings of liquid polish on your nails?"*: Antoinette Donnelly, "Our Best Manicure Circles Put Ban on the Double Shine," *Chicago Daily Tribune*, September 25, 1925, p. 28.

165 *"There seems to be some doubt in the minds of a great many women"*: Viola Paris, "Beauty and You: Liquid Nail Polish," *Washington Post*, December 22, 1926, p. 12 (syndicated by *Vogue*); Lydia Lane, "Care of Nails Beauty Need: Cracking Blamed of Use of Liquid Polish," *Los Angeles Times*, December 31, 1935, p. A7.

165 *"purplish, brownish or bluish color"*: Viola Paris, "Beauty and You: Little Tips about Nails," *Washington Post*, March 4, 1927, p. 12; Lydia Lane, "Massage and Oil Develop Unbreakable Finger Nails: Beauty Authority Tells of Preparation to Prevent Exclamation of Regret," *Los Angeles Times*, May 2, 1935, p. A5.

166 *"Finger nails tinted, enameled and polished to match one's pearl necklace"*: Anon., "Tinted Nail Is London Fad," *NYT*, September 11, 1927, p. E6; also Elsie Pierce, "How to Be Beautiful: It Takes a Beautiful Hand to Wear Jewels and High-Color Nail Polishes with an Air," *Washington Post*, June 17, 1932, p. 9; Ruth Anne Davis, "Sunset Colors Glow in Nail Polish; Mexican Trend in Merchandise," *Washington Post*, February 9, 1934, p. 12; "The Post Impressionist: Red Badge of Courage?" *Washington Post*, August 2, 1934, p. 8 (fire-alarm fingernails).

166 *"Extravagance in manicure"*: Ruth Anne Davis, "Sunset Colors Glow in Nail Polish; Mexican Trend in Merchandise," *Washington Post*, February 9, 1934, p. 12.

166 *"Queen Mary"*: Anon., "Queen Mary in '5 and 10' Shop Buys 'Thrillers' For King to Read and Nail Polish for Herself," *NYT*, February 26, 1929, p. 1 (by special cable).

167 *a rearguard action against vivid color*: Anon., "Bobbed Hair and Tinted Nails Called Self-Mutilation," *Science News-Letter*, vol. 25, no. 687, June 9, 1934, p. 364.

167 *Cutex*: Kate Forde, "Celluloid Dreams: The Marketing of Cutex in America, 1916–1935," *Journal of Design History*, vol. 15, 2002, pp. 175–89.

167 *Madame Yevonde*: (1893–1975) "Women's Passion for Colour: Mauve Hair and Bright Green Toe-Nails," *The Times*, December 7, 1932, p. 17. In Madame Yevonde's Vivex color print portraits *Viscountess Ratendone as Euterpe*, 1935, and *Gertrude Lawrence, Possibly as the Muse of Comedy*, 1936 (both London: National Portrait Gallery), both sitters pose with glossily polished nails—red.

167 *"nail polish which will not chip, peel, or fade"*: "Made in thirteen shades as well as colourless and natural. 1s. 6d." *The Times*, November 16, 1938, p. 19.

167 *Massy*: George Latham Massy, also of Berridge, Sunningdale, Berks., "Painted Finger-Nails: To the Editor of The Times," August 3, 1937, p. 11. See also Werner Sollors, "The Bluish Tinge in the Halfmoon; or, Fingernails as a Racial Sign," chap. 5 of his *Neither Black Nor White, Yet Both: Thematic Explorations of Interracial Literature*, Cary, N.C.: Oxford University Press, 1997, pp. 142–61. A slight variant on this unpleasant theme is found in Louis Athes's book *Lawyers and Immigrants, 1870–1940: A Cultural History*, New York: LFB Scholarly Publishing, 2003, pp. 60–61, where on Ellis Island clean, well-kept fingernails were apparently sufficient for Italian women to escape from being automatically categorized as "dagoes."

168 *R. Haslam Jackson*: Dated August 3, 1937, the letter was published two days later, under the title "Painted Finger-Nails: To the Editor of The Times," August 5, p. 11; see also "Painted Finger-Nails: To the Editor of The Times," August 27, 1937, p. 8. For the gilded nails of the ancient Egyptians, see Aviva Briefel, "Hands of Beauty, Hands of Horror: Fear and Egyptian Art at the Fin de Siècle," *Victorian Studies*, vol. 50, no. 2 (Winter 2008): pp. 263–71.

169 *"fashionable French resort"*: Michael Burn, "Painted Finger-Nails: To the Editor of The Times," August 6, 1937, p. 13.

169 *"Lady Mary Wortley Montagu"*: Arnold Hyde, of Clayton Bridge, Manchester, "Painted Finger-Nails: To the Editor of The Times," August 7, 1937, p. 11. See also the slightly different, original text of Lady Mary's letter to the Countess of Mar (April 1, 1717): Lord Wharncliffe and W. Moy Thomas, eds., *The Letters and Works of Lady Mary Wortley Montagu*, London: Henry G. Bohn, vol. 1, 1861, p. 175.

170 *Moody*: Harold Arundel Moody (1882–1947), "Painted Finger-Nails: To the Editor of The Times," August 11, 1937, p. 13.

171 *Thomas Bodkin*: "Painted Finger-Nails: To the Editor of The Times," August 18, 1937, p. 11. Thomas Patrick Bodkin (1887–1961) was a nephew of Hugh Lane; secretary to the commissioners for charitable donations and bequests, 1917–35; member of the Irish government commission on coinage, 1926; member of organizing committee of the National Museum of Ireland, 1927; director of the National Gallery of Ireland, 1927–35, and Barber Professor of Fine Arts, Barber Institute, University of Birmingham, 1935–52; *chevalier* (1933) then *officier* (1952) of the Légion d'honneur, 1933; papal knight, 1952. Georges-Charles-Nicolas-Marie Hulin de Loo (1862–1945) was a French-speaking native of Ghent, a pioneer in the systematic study of fifteenth-century Flemish paintings, sometime professor at the university and the École des Hautes Études in Ghent, as well as at the Institut supérieur d'Histoire et d'Archéologie in Brussels. He was a member of the consultative committee of the *Burlington Magazine*.

172 *"the sheep of Panurge"*: The reference here is to the story in Book IV, chap. 8, of François Rabelais's *Gargantua and Pantagruel*. At the end of the month, this sequence of correspondence prompted a comic reprise in *Time* (New York), vol. 30, no. 9, August 30, 1937: "Last week, and for a fortnight before ... [*The Times's*] volunteer correspondents were engaged in a controversy moderately scandalous for them, but they handled it with their usual decorum and historical perspective ... To the defense of his industry came R. H. Oackson [*sic*], editor of *Perfumery and Toileting* [*sic*] ... The letters were running about 50–50 on the subject when R. W. Alston, whose inquiring mind had profited by the August bank holiday offered a new idea: 'Recently I visited the seaside and was flattered to find myself the object of attentive curiosity until I realized that the ladies who met me with arched eyebrows were not surprised or delighted, but merely plucked and therefore incapable of any other expression.'"

8. The Finger of Play

177 *Song of Solomon* (King James, 1611): The Song of Solomon is accepted by many exegetes as having been composed in Hebrew at around the time of King Solomon, c. early- to mid-twentieth-century B.C.E. The Vulgate Latin text reads "*surrexi ut aperirem delicto meo manus meae stillaverunt murra* digiti mei plena murra *probatissima*" (my italics).

177 *"Bowlers with plenty of finger-spin"*: pp. 2–3. The sentence, which refers to the quintessentially English game of cricket, means: Players who bowl the ball with plenty of finger-spin are most likely to devastate the opposing team by dismissing more batsmen than if they do not.

181 *with or without spin*: See David Allen, "The Art of Spinning," in Jim Parks, ed., *The Commonwealth Book of Cricket*, London: Stanley Paul, 1963, pp. 25–28. I am indebted to Simon Trumble for clarifying several of the technical points in this section, and to our distinguished cousin Robert Trumble for his cumulative historical exegesis in *The Golden Age of Cricket*, Melbourne: Author, 1968, *passim*.

181 *Bosanquet*: Christopher Martin-Jenkins, "Bosanquet, Bernard James Tindal (1877–1936)," *The Complete Who's Who of Test Cricketers*, Adelaide: Rigby, 1980, pp. 19–20. The game of "Twisty Grab," also known as "Tishy-Toshy," is described at length by Francis Meynell, ed., *The Weekend Book*, London: Gerald Duckworth & Co., 2005, p. 146. It appears to have been a staple of Edwardian house parties, officers' messes, and cricket clubs, especially during those frequent periods when inclement weather interrupted play.

183 *the chamber music of Haydn*: William Drabkin, "Fingering in Haydn's String Quartets," *Early Music*, vol. 16, no. 1, February 1988, pp. 50–57.

183 *wind instruments*: Albert R. Rice, "Clarinet Fingering Charts, 1732–1816," *Galpin Society Journal*, vol. 37, March 1984, pp. 16–41; Bruce Haynes, "Oboe Fingering Charts, 1695–1816," *Galpin Society Journal*, vol. 31, May 1978, pp. 68–93; Paul J. White, "Early Bassoon Fingering Charts," *Galpin Society Journal*, vol. 43, March 1990, pp. 68–111.

187 *the game of love*: See Raymond Tallis, "The Carnal Hand," section 5.2 of his magisterial *The Hand: A Philosophical Inquiry into Human Being*, Edinburgh: Edinburgh University Press, 2003, pp. 135–46; Elizabeth D. Harvey, *Sensible Flesh: On Touch in Early Modern Culture*, Philadelphia: University of Pennsylvania Press, 2002; and Lina Holler, *Erotic Morality: The Role of Touch in Moral Agency*, New Brunswick, N.J.: Rutgers University Press, 2002, *passim*.

190 *Richard Heber*: Richard Heber is not to be confused with his half brother Reginald, who in later life became second Church of England bishop of Calcutta and composed the famous hymns "Holy, Holy, Holy, Lord God Almighty" and "God That Madest Earth and Heaven." Bishop Heber died while taking a bath, halfway through a pastoral visitation of South India.

9. The Finger of Combat

191 *"Blessed be the LORD my strength"*: King James, 1611, *cfr.* the note to Psalm 144:2 in Robert Alter's recent magisterial translation, in which he suggests that the reference to fingers might allude to the pulling of the archer's bowstring. *The Book of Psalms: A Translation with Commentary*, New York and London: W. W. Norton and Company, 2007, p. 495.

191 *Sei Shōnagon*: "Hateful Things," from *Makura no shōshi, The Pillow Book of Sei Shōnagon*, translated and edited by Ivan I. Morris, New York: Columbia University Press, p. 45.

191 *Daniel Farson: Never a Normal Man*, London: HarperCollins, 1997, pp. 257–58, *cit.* Martin Gayford and Karen Wright, eds., *The Penguin Book of Art Writing*, Harmondsworth: Middlesex, 1998, p. 533.

192 *"the finger"*: Jesse Sheidlower, ed., *The F Word*, New York: Random House, 1995; Roger E. Axtell, *Gestures: The Do's and Taboos of Body Language around the World*, revised and expanded ed., New York: John Wiley and Sons, 1998, pp. 30–33.

195 Driver's Manual: Ed. William K. Seymour, and published in Hartford in 1999 under the direction of José O. Salinas, State of Connecticut commissioner of the Department of Motor Vehicles, p. 62. But see Brian Bowling, "First Amendment Suit against Pittsburgh over Middle Finger Heads to U.S. Court," *Pittsburgh Tribune-Review*, Monday, September 7, 2009, apparently arising from the plucky decision of District Court judge David S. Cercone that giving someone the finger falls under the protection of the free-speech provision of the U.S. Constitution.

196 mano fica: Umiker-Sebeok and Sebeok, *Monastic Sign Languages*, pp. 20–21. This gesture was widespread, and seems to relate directly to the old English expression "not to *care* or *give a fig* for something" or "by my fig" or "figgins," or "by hard figs," or "fig's end," viz. "all these expressions . . . probably derive from the 16th century obs. Insult . . . with accompanying gesture. To 'make the Spanish fig' was to stick your thumb between the second and third fingers, with obvious sexual symbolism." Bozz.

196 *Aristophanes*: Carl A. Anderson, "Athena's Big Finger: An Unnoticed Sexual Joke in Aristophanes' Knights," *Classical Philology*, vol. 103, no. 2, April 1, 2008, pp. 175–81.

196 *and by physical restraint, because it is very difficult to move one independently of the other*: Incredibly, a surgical procedure was successfully adopted in the 1930s "in which the intertendinous bands joining the extensor tendon of the fourth finger to that of the third and of the fifth are removed" for the benefit of keyboard musicians seeking to "strengthen" the independent range of motion of the "weak" ring finger. P. R. Boucher, "Operation to Aid Fourth Finger," *The Musical Times*, October 1942, p. 31.

196 digitus medicus: Frederick Thomas Elworthy, *The Evil Eye*, London: John Murray, 1895, p. 319.

197 *Martial*: *cit.* and translated by Amy Richlin, *The Garden of Priapus: Sexuality and Aggression in Roman Humor*, New Haven: Yale University Press, 1983, p. 132: "*Rideto multum qui te, Sextille, cinaedum / dixerit et* digitum porrigito medium. / *sed nec pedico es nec tu, Sextille, fututor, / calda Vetustinae nec tibi bucca placet; / ex istis nihil es, fateor, Sextille: quid ergo es? / nescio, sed tu scis res superesse duas.*"

197 *herms and terms*: Henning Wrede, *Die antike Herme*, Mainz: Philipp von Zabern, 1986.

198 *inferences of homosexuality*: But see K. J. Dover's brilliant remarks about the occurrence in Greek vase paintings of apparently obscene gestures of pointing at the buttocks in his magisterial *Greek Homosexuality*, updated edition, Cambridge, Mass.: Harvard University Press, 1989, pp. 5ff., 92.

198 *they are nowhere any longer understood to be obscene*: See, for example, the vast range and number of pointing functions accumulated by Sotaro Kita and his colleagues in their *Pointing: Where Language, Culture, and Cognition Meet*, Mahwah, N.J., and London: Lawrence Erlbaum Associates, 2003.

198 *Carl Sittl: Die Gebärden der Griechen und Römer*, Leipzig: Teubner, 1890, p. 95.

198 *Caligula*: Suetonius, 56.

200 *chat rooms, forums, blogs, and other places on the Internet*: See for, example, the disorderly article at en.wikipedia.org/wiki/Finger_(gesture); and subsequent iterations in (a) an exchange between Adam Koford of Salt Lake City, Utah, and Cecil Adams at www.straightdope.com/columns/read/1279/whats-the-origin-of-the-finger; (b) www.ooze.com/finger/html/history.html and www.ooze.com/finger/html/foreign.html; (c) wiki.answers.com/Q/Where_does_giving_the_finger_originate_from; and (d) www.answerbag.com/q_view/61378 (all accessed April 25, 2009); the issue is also raised by innumerable bloggers.

201 *"the arts of personal combat"*: See (*inter alia*) H[enry]. B[lackwell]., *The Gentleman's Tutor for the Small Sword: or, The Compleat English Fencing Master*, London: Printed for J. and T.W., 1730; Francis Grose, *Military Antiquities Respecting a History of the English Army: From the Conquest to the Present Time*, London: Printed for S. Hooper no. 212 High Holborn, 1786–88; Captain G. Sinclair [42nd Regt.], *Cudgel-Playing Modernized and Improved; or, The Science of Defense*, London: Printed and Sold by J. Bailey, 116, Chancery-Lane, 1800; Henry C. Angelo, *Angelo's Bayonet Exercise*, London: Parker, Furnivall, and Park, Military Library, Whitehall, 1853; Lorenzo Sabine, *Notes on Duels and Duelling*, 3rd ed., Boston: Crosby, Nichols, and Co., 1859; Sir Richard F. Burton, *The Book of the Sword*, London: Chatto and Windus, 1884; Charles ffoulkes and Capt. E. C. Hopkinson, *Sword, Lance and Bayonet: A Record of the Arms of the British Army and Navy*, Cambridge: Cambridge University Press, 1938; Edmund H. Burke, *The History of Archery*, New York: Morrow, 1957; R. Ewart Oakeshott, *The Archaeology of Weapons: Arms and Armour from Prehistory to the Age of Chivalry*, London: Lutterworth Press, 1960; Robert Baldick, *The Duel: A History of Duelling*, London and New York: Spring, 1965; Frederick Wilkinson, *Small Arms*, London: Ward Lock, 1965, and his *Swords and Daggers*, London: Ward Lock, 1967; Arthur Wise, *The Art and History of Personal Combat*, Greenwich, Conn.: New York Graphic Society Ltd., 1971.

203 *gun-related deaths in America*: these figures come from the Center for Gun Policy and Research at Johns Hopkins Bloomberg School of Public Health,

www.jhsph.edu/publichealthnews/articles/2007/vernick_gun_trafficking
.html (accessed March 29, 2009).

10. The Strange Status of the Thumb

In this chapter I have been greatly assisted by W. Strickland, *The Thumb*, Edinburgh and New York: Churchill Livingstone, 1994.

207 *"By the pricking of my thumbs"*: See also W. H.-A., "Divination by Twitching," *N&Q*, 11th series, vol. 8, September 6, 1913, p. 187; L. E. Hertslet, "Folklore of the Skin," *N&Q*, September 29, 1928, p. 228; M. E. Grenander, "Macbeth IV.i.44–45 and Convulsive Ergotism," *English Language Notes*, vol. 15, 1977, pp. 102–103, where it is pluckily argued that the second witch's thumbs are pricking at Macbeth's approach because she is afflicted with ergotism or ergot blight, a disease apparently once associated with witchcraft, and apparently caused by consuming grain infested with funguses belonging to the ergot family (*gen.* Claviceps).

207 *Jacob Bronowski*: London: BBC, 1973, pp. 256–57.

211 *pediatric medicine*: Jonathan Gillis, "Bad Habits and Pernicious Results: Thumb Sucking and the Discipline of Late-Nineteenth-Century Paediatrics," *Medical History*, vol. 40, no. 1, 1996, pp. 55–73.

212 *child psychologists in Oxford*: Anon., "Conclusions on Thumb-Sucking: 'Pleasant Way of Passing Time,'" *The Times*, September 8, 1954, p. 4; Maurice D. Hart, "Thumb-Sucking," *The Times*, September 11, 1954, p. 7; E. Graham, "Thumb-Sucking," *The Times*, September 20, 1954, p. 9.

213 *our consultation with an appropriately qualified medical practitioner*: See Jerome Groopman, *How Doctors Think*, Boston: Houghton Mifflin, 2007, pp. 198–99, where some computer-generated diagnostic tools are critiqued. It is somewhat disturbing to note that Yale University now provides its graduate students with lessons in "proper handshaking technique." See Gila Reinstein, in the *Yale Bulletin and Calendar*, vol. 36, no. 13, December 14, 2007, p. 12.

214 *abnormal contractions and paralyses*: The English artist Hablot Knight Browne, known as "Phiz," who provided illustrations for many novelists, including Charles Dickens, in 1867 suffered a severe paralytic episode, maybe a stroke, that rendered his thumb useless. Nevertheless, he trained himself to draw with a pencil held between his index and middle fingers, and used his limp and unopposable thumb for rubbing and shading with "housemaids' black-lead." See Robert L. Patten and Valerie Browne Lester's article in *ODNB*, vol. 8, pp. 167–68. It seems that following "an illness," the distinguished doctor Sir Rutherford Alcock (1809–97) suffered from a similar form of paralysis of both thumbs, and upon reflection wisely abandoned his busy surgical practice in favor of diplomacy. See M. H. Kaufman, "The Military Career of Mr. (Later Sir) Rutherford Alcock (1809–97)," *Journal of Medical Biography*, vol. 13, no. 1, 2005, pp. 3–10.

214 *The hand and the fingers as diagnostic tools*: See Markwart Michler, *Die Hand als Werkzeug des Arztes: Eine kurze Geschichte der Palpation von den Anfängen bis zur Gegenwart* (Beiträge zur Geschichte der Wissenschaft und der Technik, 12), Wiesbaden: Franz Steiner Verlag, 1972.

215 *the seer and the doctor in antiquity*: See K. Gross, "Finger," in Theodor Klauser, ed., *Reallexikon für Antike und Christentum*, vol. 7, Stuttgart: Anton Hiersemann, 1968, pp. 909–46, and Michael Attyah Flower, *The Seer in Ancient Greece*, Berkeley, Calif.: University of California Press, 2008, pp. 8, 25, 130–31 (re. "Hepatoscopy," or the careful inspection of livers).

215 *Leopold Auenbrugger: Novum Inventum ex Percussione Thoracis Humani.* Vienna: Joannis Thomae Trattner, 1761; see also Saul Jarcho, "A Review of Auenbrugger's *Inventum Novum*, Attributed to Oliver Goldsmith [in the *Public Ledger*, August 27, 1761]," *Bulletin of the History of Medicine*, vol. 33, September–October 1959, pp. 470–74; Saul Jarcho, "[Giovanni Battista] Morgagni and Auenbrugger in the Retrospect of Two Hundred Years," *Bulletin of the History of Medicine*, vol. 35, no. 6, November–December 1961, pp. 489–96; D. Evan Bedford, "Auenbrugger's Contribution to Cardiology: History of Percussion of the Heart," *British Heart Journal*, vol. 33, 1971, pp. 817–21; Malcolm Nicolson, "The Introduction of Percussion and Stethoscopy to Early Nineteenth-Century Edinburgh," in W. F. Bynum and Roy Porter, eds., *Medicine and the Five Senses*, Cambridge: Cambridge University Press, 1993, pp. 134–53; John C. O'Neal, "Auenbrugger, Corvisart, and the Perception of Disease," *Eighteenth-Century Studies*, vol. 31, 1998, pp. 473–89, and O. R. McCarthy, "Getting a Feel for Percussion," *Vesalius: Acta internationalis historiae medicinae*, vol. 5, no. 1, June 1999, pp. 3–10.

217 *Bartol: The Rising Faith*, Boston: Roberts Brothers, 1874, p. 175.

218 *two fingers*: Anon., "Two Fingers," *Saturday Review*, September 12, 1863, vol. 16, no. 411, p. 349. "Led captain" means "An obsequious person, who dances attendance on the master and mistress of a house, for which service he has a knife and fork at the dinner table. He is led like a dog, and always graced with the title of captain." Brewer.

219 *the gesture of "thumbs down"*: See Anthony Corbeill, "Thumbs in Ancient Rome: *Pollex* as Index," *Memoirs of the American Academy in Rome*, vol. 42, 1997, 61–81; Anthony Corbeill, "The Power of Thumbs," chap. 2 of his *Nature Embodied: Gesture in Ancient Rome*, Princeton, N.J.: Princeton University Press, 2004, pp. 41–66.

219 *Juvenal: Satires*, 3:36.

219 *Quintilian: Institutio Oratoria*, 11:3:119.

220 *collection of stray poems*: *Anthologia Latina*, 415:27–28.

220 *Pliny: Natural History*, 28:25.

Further Reading

1. A note on sources and the Internet; 2. General; 3. Finger words; 4. The finger of God; 5. Touch; 6. The fingers and finger habits of infants and children; 7. Diseases, injuries, and disabilities; 8. Polydactyly; 9. Finger mutilation; 10. Counting, and finger games; 11. Prehistoric hand images; 12. The finger in later art; 13. Gesture in culture; 14. Ancient Near Eastern, Greco-Roman, and early Christian gesture; 15. Renaissance-to-eighteenth-century gesture; 16. African gesture; 17. Asian, Oceanic, and Meso-American gesture; 18. Gesture and obscenity; 19. Sign languages; 20. Manners; 21. Fingernails; 22. Finger rings; 23. Fingerprints; 24. The signature and handwriting; 25. Gloves; 26. The finger and domestic industry; 27. The finger in drama, music, and dance; 28. The fingers in hand-to-hand combat; 29. Fingers and tobacco.

1. A note on sources and the Internet

Many of the articles and more recent books listed here were found by means of powerful search engines, indices, and other Internet resources, but not all. The sheer Niagara of apparently pertinent references is at best awkward to manage and, in the case of thousands upon thousands of "hits," overwhelming and counterproductive. True, the rapid progress that is just now being made toward the digitization of tens of thousands of old books is transforming our capacity to search for otherwise fugitive terms and concepts such as "filbert nails," for which the Victorians exhibited such a bafflingly persistent taste. Yet in most departments I have found it best to persist with those woolly mammoths *The British Library General Catalogue of Printed Books to 1975* (366 vols., London, Munich, New York, and Paris: K. G. Saur, 1979–1987) and the Library of Congress's even more enormous 754-volume *The National Union Catalog: Pre-1956 Imprints* (Chicago and London: Mansell, 1968–1981), which, reproducing the old cards (together with invaluable penciled corrections, and the occasional flash of inspired marginal comment from now forgotten nineteenth- and twentieth-century librarian-sibyls), never fail to yield treasure. I dreaded the day when those volumes would be carted off to the knackers' yard, and now I am sad to say that day has finally come.

In any case, thanks to the Sterling Memorial Library; and through the Reference Library of the Yale Center for British Art, I have harnessed a number of especially astonishing search engines that still make possible the serendipitous discoveries that more often used to occur in the stacks. Most good research libraries will provide access to all of them:

Anthropological Index Online, the Anthropology Library at the British Museum, aio .anthropology.org.uk

Bibliography of Asian Studies, Association for Asian Studies, www.aasianst.org

The Bibliography of the History of Art (BHA), the J. Paul Getty Trust Art History Information Program (AHIP) and the Institut de l'Information Scientifique et Technique (INIST) of the Centre National de la Recherche Scientifique, www.rlg.org

Database of Classical Bibliography (L'Année philologique), the Société Internationale de Bibliographie Classique, the American Philological Association and the Database of Classical Bibliography, the Centre National de la Recherche Scientifique, and the National Endowment for Humanities, www.annee-philologique.com

The Dictionary of Art, Macmillan Reference and Grove's Dictionaries, Inc., www .groveart.com

Early English Books Online (EEBO), the University of Michigan, Oxford University, and ProQuest Information and Learning Company, eebo.chadwyck.com

Historical Newspapers Online, Chadwyck Healey, historynews.chadwyck.com (see also *Times Digital Archive*)

New Testament Abstracts, ATLA and the Weston Jesuit School of Theology (EBSCO Host Research Databases), www.atla.com

New York Times Historical, ProQuest Information and Learning Company, www .nyt.ulib.org

Nineteenth-Century British Newspapers Online, British Library and Gale, www .bl.uk/collections/britishnewspapers1800to1900.html

Notes and Queries, Oxford University Press, nq.oxfordjournals.org

Old Testament Abstracts Online, ATLA and the Catholic Biblical Association (EBSCO Host Research Databases), www.atla.com

Ovid, Ovid Technologies, Inc., providing access to *Evidence Based Medicine Reviews* and sundry medical and scientific indices and research databases, www.ovid.com

Oxford Dictionary of National Biography, Oxford University Press, www.oxforddnb.com

Oxford English Dictionary, Oxford University Press, www.oed.com

The Proceedings of the Old Bailey, London, 1674 to 1834, Humanities Research Institute, University of Sheffield, University of Michigan, Harvester Microform, and ProQuest Information and Learning Company as part of *Early English Books Online*, www.oldbaileyonline.org

Times Digital Archive, Thomson Gale, www.gale.com/Times

Victorian Database Online, Litir Database, Inc., www.victoriandatabase.com

2. General

David F. Armstrong, *Original Signs: Gesture, Sign, and the Sources of Language*. Washington, D.C.: Gallaudet University Press, 1999.

Eve Arnold, *Handbook (with Footnotes)*. London: Bloomsbury, 2004.

Denis Guedj, *Numbers: The Universal Language*, translated by Lory Frankel. New York: Harry N. Abrams, 1997.

Guido H. G. Joachim, *International Bibliography of Sign Language* (International Studies on Sign Language and Communication of the Deaf, 21). Hamburg: Signum Verlag, 1993.

William Jones, *Finger-Ring Lore: Historical, Legendary, Anecdotal*, 2nd rev. ed. London: Chatto and Windus, 1890.

John Manning, *The Finger Book: Sex, Behaviour and Disease Revealed in the Fingers*. London: Faber and Faber, 2008.

Howard Poizner, *What the Hands Reveal about the Brain*. Cambridge, Mass.: MIT Press, 1987.

James W. Strickland and Thomas Graham, *The Hand*, 2nd ed. Philadelphia: Lippincott and Wilkins, 2005.

Raymond Tallis, *The Hand: A Philosophical Inquiry into Human Being*. Edinburgh: Edinburgh University Press, 2003.

3. Finger words

Richard Allsopp, ed., *Dictionary of Caribbean English Usage*. Oxford: Oxford University Press, 1996.

Lester V. Berry and Melvin van den Bark, *The American Thesaurus of Slang, with Supplement: A Complete Reference Book of Colloquial Speech*. New York: Thomas Y. Cromwell Company, 1942.

"Ducange Anglicus" (pseud.), *The vulgar tongue: a glossary of slang, cant, and flash words and phrases, used in London from 1839 to 1859; flash songs, essays on slang, and a bibliography of canting and slang literature*, 2nd ed. London: B. Quaritch, 1859.

John Stephen Farmer and W. E. Henley, *Slang and its analogues, past and present. A dictionary, historical and comparative, of the heterodox speech of all classes of society for more than three hundred years, with synonyms in English, French, German, Italian, etc.* (1890–1904), 7 vols. New York: Kraus Reprint Corp., 1965.

J[ohn]. C[amden]. Hotten, *Dictionary of Modern Slang, Cant, and Vulgar Words, used at the present day in the streets of London; the universities of Oxford and Cambridge; the houses of Parliament; the dens of St. Giles; and the palaces of St. James; preceded by a history of cant*. London: J. C. Hotten, 1859.

Mary Marshall, *Bozzimacoo: Origins & Meanings of Oaths & Swear Words*. Walton-on-Thames and London: M. & J. Hobbs, in association with Michael Joseph, 1975.

Henry Mayhew, *London labour and the London poor: the condition and earnings of those that will work, cannot work, and will not work*, 3 vols. London: Charles Griffin and Co., 1951.

Eric Partridge, *A Dictionary of Slang and Unconventional English from the Fifteenth Century to the Present Day*, 5th ed. New York: Macmillan, 1961.

———, *A Dictionary of the Underworld, British and American, Being the Vocabularies of Crooks, Criminals, Racketeers, Beggars and Tramps, Convicts, the Commercial Underworld, the Drug Traffic, the White Slave Traffic, Spivs*, 3rd ed. London: Routledge & Kegan Paul, 1968.

W. S. Ramson, ed., *The Australian National Dictionary*. Melbourne: Oxford University Press, 1988.

J[ames]. Redding Ware, *Passing English of the Victorian era, a dictionary of heterodox English, slang, and phrase*. London: G. Routledge & Sons, 1909.

Ernest Weekley, *Etymological Dictionary of Modern English*. London: John Murray, 1921.

Joseph Wright, *English Dialect Dictionary: Being the complete vocabulary of all dialect words still in use, or known to have been in use during the last two hundred years*. London: Henry Frowde, 1905.

4. The finger of God

P. W. van der Horst, "'The Finger of God' (Miscellaneous Notes on Luke 11:20) and Its *Umwelt*," in W. L. Petersen et al., eds., *Sayings of Jesus: Canonical and Non-Canonical: Essays in Honor of Tjitze Baarda* (Supplements to Novum Testamentum, 89). Leiden and New York: Brill, 1997, pp. 89–103.

G. A. Klingbeil, "The Finger of God in the Old Testament," *Zeitschrift für die Alttestamentliche Wissenschaft*, vol. 112, no. 3, 2000, pp. 409–15.

Scott B. Noegel, "Moses and Magic: Notes on the Book of Exodus," *Journal of the Ancient Near Eastern Society*, vol. 24, 1996, pp. 45–59.

L. Perkins, "Why the 'Finger of God' in Luke 11:20," *Expository Times*, vol. 115, no. 8 (2004), pp. 261–62.

Joseph Reindl, "Der Finger Gottes und die Macht der Götter," in Wilhelm Ernst, ed., *Dienst der Vermittlung: Festschrift zum 25-jährigen Bestehen des Philosoph-Theologischen Studiums Erfurt* (Erfurter Theologische Studien, 37), Leipzig: St. Benno, 1977, pp. 49–60.

R. W. Wall, "'The Finger of God': Deuteronomy 9.10 and Luke 11.20," *New Testament Studies*, vol. 33, no. 1 (1987), pp. 144–50.

E. J. Woods, *The "Finger of God" and Pneumatology in Luke–Acts* (JSNT Supplement Series, 205). Sheffield, England: Sheffield Academic Press, 2001.

5. Touch

Elizabeth D. Harvey, *Sensible Flesh: On Touch in Early Modern Culture*. Philadelphia: University of Pennsylvania Press, 2002.

Lina Holler, *Erotic Morality: The Role of Touch in Moral Agency*. New Brunswick, N.J.: Rutgers University Press, 2002.

Dominick Leupold-Kirschneck, *Das Handauflegen: Eine ärztliche Urgebärbe in Geschichte und Gegenwart*. Basel: Schwarbe, 1981.

Ashley Montagu, *Touching: The Human Significance of the Skin*. New York: Harper & Row, 1977.

Micla Petrelli et al., *Valori tattili e arte del sensibile*. Florence: Alinea, 1994.

Yngve Zotterman, *Touch, Tickle, and Pain*, 2 vols. Oxford and New York: Pergamon Press, 1969–71.

6. The fingers and finger habits of infants and children

Lucille H. Blum and Anna Dragositz, "Finger Painting: The Developmental Aspects," *Child Development*, vol. 18, no. 3 (September 1947), pp. 88–105.

L. C. Breen, "Diagnosis of Behavior by Finger Painting," *Elementary School Journal*, vol. 56, no. 7 (March 1956), pp. 321–24.

Jonathan Gillis, "Bad Habits and Pernicious Results: Thumb Sucking and the Discipline of Late-Nineteenth-Century Paediatrics," *Medical History*, vol. 40, no. 1 (1996), pp. 55–73.

Mary Sakraida Kunst, *A Study of Thumb- and Finger-Sucking in Infants* (Psychological Monographs: General and Applied, 290). Washington, D.C.: American Psychological Association, 1948.

Arthur Lefford, "The Perceptual and Cognitive Bases for Finger Localization and Selective Finger Movement in Preschool Children," *Child Development*, vol. 45, no. 2 (June 1974), pp. 335–43.

David M. Levy, "Thumb or Fingersucking from the Psychiatric Angle," *Child Development*, vol. 8, no. 1 (March 1937), pp. 99–101.

Iris McGuire and Gerald Turkewitz, "Visually Elicited Finger Movements in Infants," *Child Development*, vol. 49, no. 2 (June 1978), pp. 362–70.

James C. Reed, "Lateralized Finger Agnosia and Reading Achievement at Ages 6 and 10," *Child Development*, vol. 38, no. 1 (March 1967), pp. 213–20.

Ruth Staples and Helen Conley, "The Use of Color in the Finger Painting of Young Children," *Child Development*, vol. 20, no. 4 (December 1949), pp. 201–12.

Ames F. Tryon, "Thumb-Sucking and Manifest Anxiety: A Note," *Child Development*, vol. 39, no. 4 (December 1968), pp. 1159–63.

7. *Diseases, injuries, and disabilities*
Peter Brüser and Alain Gilbert, *Finger Bone and Joint Injuries*. London: Martin Dunitz, 1999.

D. A. Campbell-Reid and D. A. McGrouther, *Surgery of the Thumb*. London and Boston: Butterworths, 1986.

Condict Walker Cutler, *The Hand, Its Disabilities and Diseases*. Philadelphia: W. B. Saunders Company, 1942.

Karl M. Dallenbach, "A Comparative Study of the Errors of Localization on the Finger-Tips," *American Journal of Psychology*, vol. 44, no. 2 (April 1932), pp. 327–31.

Julien Glicenstein, *Tumours of the Hand*, translated by David LeVay. Berlin and New York: Springer Verlag, 1988.

H. Kelikian, *Congenital Deformities of the Hand and Forearm*. Philadelphia: W. B. Saunders Company, 1974.

A. Landi et al., eds., *Reconstruction of the Thumb*. London: Chapman and Hall, 1989.

Charles T. Price, *Pediatric Upper Extremity Fractures*. Rosemont, Ill.: American Academy of Orthopedic Surgeons, 2004.

Elden C. Weckesser, *Treatment of Hand Injuries: Preservation and Restoration of Function*. Chicago: Year Book Medical Publishers, 1974.

8. *Polydactyly*
Richard D. Barnett, "Six Fingers and Six Toes: Polydactylism in the Ancient World," *Biblical Archaeology Review*, vol. 16, no. 3 (1990), pp. 46–51.

———, "Six Fingers in Art and Archaeology," *Bulletin of the Anglo-Israel Archaeological Society*, vol. 6 (1986–87), pp. 5–12.

Walter Blauth, *Congenital Deformities of the Hand*, translated by U. H. Weil. Berlin and New York: Springer Verlag, 1981.

Sir Anthony Carlisle, *An Account of a Family Having Hands and Feet with Supernumary Fingers and Toes . . . In a Letter Addressed to Sir Joseph Banks . . . Read December 23, 1813*. London, off-printed from *Philosophical Transactions*, 1814.

Adrian E. Flatt, *The Care of Congenital Hand Anomalies*, 2nd ed. St. Louis, Mo.: Quality Medical Pub., 1994.

Armand Marie Leroi, *Mutants: On Genetic Variety and the Human Body*. New York: Viking Penguin, 2003.

Hildegard Urner-Astholz, "Sechs Finger und sechs Zehen in der mittelalterlichen Symbolik," *Zeitschrift für schweizerische Archäologie und Kunstgeschichte*, vol. 54 (1997), pp. 329–36.

9. Finger mutilation

Neil McLeod, "Compensation for Fingers and Teeth in Early Irish Law," *Peritia: Journal of the Medieval Academy of Ireland*, vol. 16 (2002), pp. 344–59.

Lellia Cracco Ruggini, "Mutilation of the Self: Cutting Off Fingers or Ears as a Protest in Antiquity," *Atti dell'Accademia nazionale dei Lincei*, 9th series, vol. 9, no. 3 (1998), pp. 375–85.

John A. Rush, *Spiritual Tattoo: A Cultural History of Tattooing, Piercing, Scarification, Branding, and Implants*. Berkeley, Calif.: Frog, 2005.

Ali Sahly, *Les Mains mutilées dans l'art préhistorique*. Toulouse: Faculté des Lettres et Sciences Humaines de Toulouse, 1966.

John James Scanlon, *The Mutilated Hand and the Workmen's Compensation Act, 1906, Having Special Reference to "Missing" Fingers*. London: Scientific Press, 1913.

10. Counting, and finger games

Clavin C. Clawson, *The Mathematical Traveler: Exploring the Grand History of Numbers*. New York and London: Plenum Press, 1994.

Gloria T. Delamar, *Children's Counting-Out Rhymes, Fingerplays, Jump-Rope, and Bounce-Ball Chants and Other Rhymes: A Comprehensive English-Language Reference*. Jefferson, N.C.: McFarland, 1983.

Graham Flegg, *Numbers: Their History and Meaning*. New York: Schocken Books, 1983.

Alexander Humez et al., *Zero to Lazy Eight: The Romance of Numbers*. New York: Simon and Schuster, 1993.

Georges Ifrah, *The Universal History of Numbers*, translated by David Bellos, E. F. Harding, et al., 3 vols. London: Harvill, 2000.

Aaron Logg, "Fists, Fingers and Figures, The Natural Abacus," in *Crossed Hands; or Logg's Logical Arithmetic*. London: privately printed, 1911.

Brian Rotman, *Mathematics as Sign: Writing, Imagining, Counting*. Stanford, Calif.: Stanford University Press, 2000.

11. Prehistoric hand images

Claude Barrière, *L'Art pariétal de la Grotte de Gargas*, translated by W. A. Drapkin. Oxford: British Archaeological Reports, 1976.

Harold Cummins, "The 'Finger-Print' Carvings of Stone-Age Men in Brittany," *The Scientific Monthly*, vol. 31, no. 3 (September 1930), pp. 273–79.

Robert Layton, *Australian Rock Art: A New Synthesis*. Cambridge: Cambridge University Press, 1992.

W. C. McGrew et al., "Thumbs, Tools, and Early Humans," *Science*, n.s., vol. 268, no. 5210 (April 28, 1995), pp. 586–89.

Jacques Pelegrin, "La Main et l'outil préhistorique," in *La Main* (Eurasie: Cahiers de la Société des Études euro-asiatiques, 4). Paris: Editions L'Harmattan, 1993, pp. 19–25.

A. R. Verbrugge, *Corpus of the Hand Figurations in Primitive Australia*. Compiègne: Éditions Orphrys, 1970.

———, *Le Symbole de la main dans la préhistoire*. New and expanded ed. Compiègne: Author, 1969.

12. The finger in later art

Suzanne Preston Blier, *Gestures in African Art*. New York: L. Kahan Gallery, 1982.

Richard Brilliant, *Gesture and Rank in Roman Art: The Use of Gestures to Denote Status in Roman Sculpture and Coinage*. New Haven: Connecticut Academy of Arts and Sciences, 1963.

Heinz Demisch, *Erhobene Hände: Geschichte einer Gebärde in der bildenden Kunst*. Stuttgart: Urachhaus, 1984.

Brigitte Dominicus, *Gesten und Gebärden in Darstellungen des Altes und Mittleren Reiches* (Studien zur Archäologie und Geschichte Altägyptens, 10). Heidelberg: Heidelberger Orientverlag, 1994.

Hilde Frauender et al., *Beredete Hände: Die Bedeutung von Gesten in der Kunst des 16. Jahrhunderts bis zur Gegenwart*. Salzburg: Residenzgalerie, 2004.

Suzanne Karr, "Constructions Both Sacred and Profane: Serpents, Angels, and Pointing Fingers in Renaissance Books with Moving Parts," *Yale University Library Gazette*, vol. 78, nos. 3–4 (2004), pp. 101–27.

Liselore Kirchner, *Jungpaläolithische Handdarstellungen der franko-kantabrischen Felsbilderzone: ein Versuch ihrer Deutung unter Berücksichtigung ethnographischer Parallelen*. Göppingen: Druck Werner-Müller, 1959.

Timothy McNiven, "Gestures in Attic Vase Painting: Use and Meaning, 550–450 B.C." University of Michigan Ph.D. dissertation, 1982.

Michel Merle et al., *Rodin, les mains, les chirurgiens*. Paris: Musée Rodin, 1983.

John Murphy, "Gesture, Magic, and Primitive Art," *Man*, vol. 40 (August 1940), pp. 119–21.

Ljiljana Ortolja-Baird, ed., *Hands in Art*. London and New York: Bridgeman Art Library, 2000.

Ulrich Rehm, *Stumme Sprache der Bilder: Gestik als Mittel neuzeitlicher Bilderzählung*. Munich: Deutscher Kunstverlag, 2002.

Klaas Ruitenbeek, *Discarding the Brush: Gao Qipei (1660–1734) and the Art of Chinese Finger Painting*, with an essay by Joan Stanley-Baker. Ghent: Snoeck-Ducaju and Zoon, 1992.

———, "Jenseits von Pinsel und Tusche: Fingermalerei in Ostasien und Europa," *Monumenta Serica*, vol. 49 (2001), pp. 445–62.

Trude S. Waehner, "Interpretation of Spontaneous Drawings and Paintings," *Genetic Psychology Monographs*, vol. 33 (1946), pp. 3–70.

Michaela Walliser-Wurster, *Fingerzeige: Studien zu Bedeutung und Funktion Geste in der bildenden Kunst der italienischen Renaissance*. Frankfurt am Main: Peter Lang, 2001.

13. Gesture in culture

Tiziana Baldizzone et al., *La Main qui parle*. Paris: Phébus, 2002.

Betty J. Bäuml and Franz H. Bäuml, *Dictionary of Worldwide Gestures*, 2nd ed. Lanham, Md., and London: Scarecrow Press, 1997.

Sergio Bertelli and Monica Centanni, eds., *Il gesto: nel rito e nel ceremoniale dal mondo antico ad oggi*. Florence: Ponte all grazie, 1995.

Jan Bremmer and Herman Roodenburg, eds., *A Cultural History of Gesture*. Ithaca, N.Y.: Cornell University Press, 1992.

Lewis Dayton Burdick, *The Hand: A Survey of Facts, Legends, and Beliefs Pertaining to Manual Ceremonies, Covenants, and Symbols*, Oxford, N.Y.: Irving Company, 1905.

C. Chambers and K. Craig, "Similarities and Differences between Cultures in Expressive Movements," in R. Hinde, ed., *Non-Verbal Communication*. Cambridge: Cambridge University Press, 1972, pp. 297–314.

Margreth Egidi et al., eds., *Gestik: Figuren des Körpers in Text und Bild* (Literatur und Anthropologie im Auftrag des Sonderforschungs-bereichs 511, 8). Tübingen: Gunter Narr Verlag, 2000.

Hanna Jursch, *Hände als Symbol und Gestalt*. Berlin: Evanelische Verlagsanstalt, 1951.

Sotaro Kita, ed., *Pointing: Where Language, Culture, and Cognition Meet*. Mahwah, N.J., and London: Lawrence Erlbaum Associates, 2003.

Jean-Hubert Levame, "Main-objet et main-image," in *La Main* (Eurasie: Cahiers de la Société des Études euro-asiatiques, 4). Paris: Editions L'Harmattan, 1993, pp. 9–18.

Johannes Maas, "Der Ausdruck der Hände; ein Beitrag zur Physiognomik der Hand und der Hände." University of Bonn "inaugural" dissertation, 1941.

David McNeill, *Hand and Mind: What Gestures Reveal about Thought*. Chicago: Chicago University Press, 1992.

Desmond Morris, *Bodytalk: A World Guide to Gestures*. London: Jonathan Cape, 1994.

——— et al., *Gestures: Their Origin and Distribution*. London: Jonathan Cape, 1979.

Jean-Claude Schmitt, ed., *Gestures*. London: Harwood Academic Publishers, 1984.

Philippe Seringe, "Symbolisme de la main," in *La Main* (Eurasie: Cahiers de la Société des Études euro-asiatiques, 4). Paris: Editions L'Harmattan, 1993, pp. 45–54.

John Wesley, *Directions concerning Pronunciation and Gesture*. Bristol: Printed by William Pine, 1770.

14. Ancient Near Eastern, Greco-Roman, and early Christian gesture

Gregory S. Aldrete, *Gestures and Acclamations in Ancient Rome*. Baltimore, Md.: Johns Hopkins University Press, 1999.

Kathrin Bogen, *Gesten in Begrüssungsszenen auf attischen Vasen*. Bonn: Rudolf Habelt Verlag, 1969.

Anthony Corbeill, *Nature Embodied: Gesture in Ancient Rome*. Princeton, N.J.: Princeton University Press, 2004.

Antonio Donghi, *Actions and Words: Symbolic Language and the Liturgy*, translated by William McDonagh and Dominic Serra. Collegeville, Minn.: Liturgical Press, 1997.

Howard Jacobson, "The Position of the Fingers during the Priestly Blessing," *Revue de Qumran*, vol. 34 (1977), pp. 259–60.

Martin Kirigin, O.S.B., *La mano divina nell'iconografia cristiana* (Studi di antichità cristiana, 31). Rome: Pontificia Istituto di Archeologia Cristiana, 1976.

Silke Knippschild, *Drum bietet zum Bunde die Hände: Rechtssymbolische Akte in zwischenstaatlichen Beziehungen im orientalischen und griechisch-römischen Altertum* (Potsdamer altertumswissenschaftliche Beiträge, 5). Stuttgart: Steiner, 2002.

Philippe Seringe, "La Main à travers les langues latine et grecque et quelques racines indo-européennes (I.E.) concernant la main ou les mains, droite et gauche," in *La Main* (Eurasie: Cahiers de la Société des Études euroasiatiques, 4). Paris: Editions L'Harmattan, 1993, pp. 55–69.

Claude Sourdive, *La Main dans l'Égypte pharaonique: Recherches de morphologie structurale sur les objets égyptiens comportant une main*. Bern and New York: P. Lang, 1984.

15. Renaissance-to-eighteenth-century gesture

Dene Barnett, *The Art of Gesture: The Practices and Principles of 18th-century Acting*. Heidelberg: C. Winter, 1987.

Gigetta Dalli Regoli, *Il gesto e la mano: convenzione e invenzione nel linguaggio figurative fra Medioevo e Rinascimento*. Florence: Leo S. Olschki, 2000.

Anne-Marie Lecoq, "Nature et rhétorique: De l'action oratoire à l'éloquence muette (John Bulwer)," *Dix-septième siècle*, vol. 33, no. 3 (1981), pp. 265–77.

Kathryn Lynch, "'What Hands Are Here?': The Hand as Generative Symbol in *Macbeth*," *Review of English Studies*, vol. 39 (1988), pp. 29–38.

Bruno Munari, *Il dizionario dei gesti italiani*. Rome: AdnKronos, 1994.

Bruno Paura, *Comme te l'aggia dicere? Ovvero l'arte gestuale a Napoli*. Naples: Intra Moenia, 1999.

Herman Roodenburg, *The Eloquence of the Body: Perspectives on Gesture in the Dutch Republic* (Studies in Netherlandish Art and Cultural History, vol. 6). Zwolle: Waanders, 2004.

Bruno Roy, "Apropos d'un geste anti-Semite decrit par Huguccio de Pise," in *Le Geste et les gestes au Moyen Age* (*Sénéfiance*, 41). Aix-en-Provence: Université de Provence, Centre universitaire d'études et de recherches médiévales d'Aix, 1998, pp. 557–70.

Hans Peter Stein, *Symbole und Zeremoniall in deutschen Streitkraft vom 18. bis zum 20. Jahrhundert* (Entwicklung deutscher militärischer Tradition, vol. 3). Herford: E. S. Mittler, 1984

16. African gesture

Hermann Hochegger, *Le Langage gestuel en Afrique Centrale* (Publications CEEBA, 2nd series, vol. 47). Bandundu, Zaïre: Centre d'études ethnologiques, 1978.

———, *Le Langage des gestes rituals* (Publications CEEBA, second series, vols. 66–68). Bandundu, Zaïre: Centre d'études ethnologiques, 1981–83.

Viviana Paques, "La Main chez les Gnawa du Maroc," in *La Main* (Eurasie: Cahiers de la Société des Études euro-asiatiques, no. 4). Paris: Editions L'Harmattan, 1993, pp. 167–78.

Susan Vogel, *Gods of Fortune: The Cult of the Hand in Nigeria* (exhibition catalog). New York: Museum of Primitive Art, 1974.

17. Asian, Oceanic, and Meso-American gesture

Pertev Naili Boratav, "La Main dans la tradition des Turcs," in *La Main* (Eurasie: Cahiers de la Société des Études euro-asiatiques, 4). Paris: Editions L'Harmattan, 1993, pp. 141–50.

Tyra af Kleen, *Mudras auf Bali: Handhaltungen der Priester* (Kulturen der Erde, vol. 15). Hagen: Folkwang Verlag, 1923.

Samuel Martí, *Mudrã: manos simbólicas en Asia y América*. Mexico City: Litexa, 1971.

Tara Michael, "Les Gestes des mains dans le ritual et dans les danses de l'Inde," in *La Main* (Eurasie: Cahiers de la Société des Études euro-asiatiques, 4). Paris: Editions L'Harmattan, 1993, pp. 91–108.

Ingrid Ramm-Bonwitt, *Mudras: Geheimsprache der Yogis*. Augsberg: Bechtermunz, 2000.

Rita H. Regnier, "Les Mains du Bouddha dans la légende et dans l'iconographie de l'Inde ancienne," in *La Main* (Eurasie: Cahiers de la Société des Études euro-asiatiques, 4). Paris: Editions L'Harmattan, 1993, pp. 109–39.

18. Gesture and obscenity

M. Caldwell, *A Short History of Rudeness: Manners, Morals, and Misbehavior in Modern America*. New York: Picador USA, 1999.

Havelock Ellis, *The Revaluation of Obscenity*. Paris: Hours Press, 1931.

Pamela Church Gibson, ed., *Dirty Looks: Gender, Pornography and Power*. London: British Film Institute, 1993.

Nicola McDonald, ed., *Medieval Obscenities*. Woodbridge, Suffolk, and Rochester, N.Y.: York Medieval, 2006.

Jesse Sheidlower, ed., *The F Word*, with a foreword by Roy Blount, Jr., 2nd ed. New York: Random House, 1999.

19. Sign languages

Robert A. Barakat, *The Cistercian Sign Language: A Study in Non-Verbal Communication*. Kalamazoo, Mich.: Cistercian Publications, 1975.

Maryse Bézagu-Deluy, *L'Abbé de l'Epée: instituteur gratuit des sourds et muets, 1712– 1789*. Paris: Seghers, 1990.

Danielle Bouvet, "L'Approche des configurations de la main dans les langues gestuelles selon des critères articulatoires," in *La Main* (Eurasie: Cahiers de la Société des Études euro-asiatiques, 4). Paris: Editions L'Harmattan, 1993, pp. 27–44.

D. Givens, "The Big and the Small: Toward a Paleontology of Gesture," *Sign Language Studies*, vol. 51 (1986), pp. 145–70.

Renate Fischer and Harlan Lane, eds., *Looking Back: A Reader on the History of Deaf Communities and Their Sign Languages* (International Studies on Sign Language and Communication of the Deaf, 20). Hamburg: Signum Verlag, 1993.

Mary E. Hazard, *Elizabethan Silent Language*. Lincoln, Neb.: University of Nebraska Press, 2000.

Cecil Lucas, ed., *Pinky Extension and Eye Gaze: Language Use in Deaf Communities* (Sociolinguistics in Deaf Communities series, 4). Washington, D.C.: Gallaudet University Press, 1998.

———, ed., *Turn-Taking, Fingerspelling and Contact in Signed Languages*. Washington, D.C.: Gallaudet University Press, 2002.

William C. Stokoe, *Language in Hand: Why Sign Came before Speech*. Washington, D.C.: Gallaudet University Press, 2001.

Jean Umiker-Sebeok and Thomas A. Sebeok, *Monastic Sign Languages* (Approaches to Semiotics, vol. 76). Berlin, Amsterdam, and New York: Mouton de Gruyter & Co., 1987.

20. Manners

F. Baldwin, *Sumptuary Legislation and Personal Regulation in England*. Baltimore, Md.: Johns Hopkins Press, 1926.

H. Baudrillart, *Histoire du luxe public et privé de l'antiquité jusqu'à nos jours*. Paris: Hachette et Cie., 1880.

E. Cooper, "Chinese Table Manners: You Are *How* You Eat," *Human Organisation*, vol. 45 (1986), pp. 179–84.

M. Curtin, "A Question of Manners: Status and Gender in Etiquette and Courtesy," *Journal of Modern History*, vol. 57 (1985), pp. 395–423.

N. Elias, *The History of Manners*, translated by Edmund Jephcott. New York: Pantheon Books, 1978.

P. Langford, *Englishness Identified: Manners and Character, 1650–1850*. Oxford: Oxford University Press, 2000.

Claude Lévi-Strauss, *The Origin of Table Manners*, translated by J. and D. Weightman. New York: Harper & Row, 1978.

Maurice J. Quinlan, *Victorian Prelude: A History of English Manners, 1700–1830*. Hamden, Conn.: Archon Books, 1965.

Margaret Visser, *The Rituals of Dinner: The Origins, Evolution, Eccentricities, and Meaning of Table Manners*. New York: Grove Weidenfeld, 1991.

21. Fingernails

M. Angeloglou, *A History of Make-Up*. London: Studio Vista, 1970.

M. Chandra, "Cosmetics and Coiffure in Ancient India," *Journal of the Indian Society of Oriental Art*, vol. 8 (1940), pp. 62–145.

M. DeNavarre, *The Chemistry and Manufacture of Cosmetics*. Orlando, Fla.: Continental Press, 1975.

J. Dixon, "Japanese Etiquette," *Transactions of the Asiatic Society of Japan*, vol. 13 (1885), pp. 1–21.

N. Etcoff, *Beauty*. New York: Doubleday, 1998.

Elisa Ferri and Lisa Kenny, with Dana Epstein, *Style on Hand: Perfect Nail and Skin Care*. New York: Universe Publishing (Rizzoli), 1998.

S. B. Finesinger, "The Customs of Looking at the Fingernails at the Outgoing of the Sabbath," in Joseph Gutmann, ed., *Beauty in Holiness: Studies in Jewish Customs and Ceremonial Art*. New York: Ktav Publishing House, 1970, pp. 262ff.

D. Laba, *Rheological Properties of Cosmetics and Toiletries*. New York: Marcel Dekker, 1993.

H. Rubinstein, *My Life for Beauty*. New York: Simon and Schuster, 1963.

Jogendra Saksena, *Art of Rajasthan: Henna and Floor Decorations*. Delhi: Sundeep, 1979.

Aline Tauzin, *Le Henné, art des femmes de Mauritanie*. Paris: Ibis Press (UNESCO), 1998.

Max Wykes-Joyce, *Cosmetics and Adornment*. New York: Philosophical Society, 1961.

22. Finger rings

Heinz Battke, *Geschichte des Ringes, in Beschreibung und Bildern*. Baden-Baden: Klein, 1953.

British Museum, *Franks Bequest: Catalogue of the Finger Rings, Early Christian, Byzantine, Teutonic, Mediaeval, and Later*. London: British Museum, 1912.

Anna Beatriz Chadour-Sampson, *Antike Fingerringe: Die Sammlung Alain Ollivier*. Munich: Prähistorische Staatssammlung München, Museum für Vor- und Frühgeschichte, 1997.

Charles Edwards, *The History and Poetry of Finger-Rings*. New York: Redfield, 1855.

George Frederick Kunz, *Rings for the Finger, from Earliest Known Times, to the Present, with full descriptions of the Origin, Early Making, Materials, the Archaeology, History, for Affection, Love, for Engagement, for Wedding, Commemorative, Mourning, etc.* Philadelphia: J. B. Lippincott Company, 1917.

Sylvie Lambert, *The Ring*. New York: Todtri, 1998.

Joseph Maskell, *The Wedding-Ring: Its History, Literature, and the Superstitions Respecting it*. London: William Freeman, 1868.

George Monger, "Rings, Wedding and Betrothal," in *Marriage Customs of the World: From Henna to Honeymoons*. Santa Barbara, Calif.: ABC-CLIO, 2004.

Diana Scarisbrick, *Rings: Symbols of Wealth, Power, and Affection*. New York: Abrams, 1993.

Anne Ward, *The Ring, from Antiquity to the Twentieth Century*. London: Thames and Hudson, 1981.

23. Fingerprints

Paul Åström and Sven A. Eriksson, *Fingerprints and Archaeology* (Studies in Mediterranean Archaeology, 28). Göteborg, Sweden: Åströms Forlag, 1980.

Harold Cummins and Charles Midlo, *Finger Prints, Palms and Soles: An Introduction to Dermatoglyphics*. New York: Dover Publications, 1961.

———— and Rebecca Wright Kennedy, "Pukinje's Observations (1823) on Finger Prints and Other Skin Features," *Journal of Criminal Law and Criminology*, vol. 31, no. 3 (September–October 1940), pp. 343–56.

Henry Pelouze DeForest, *The Evolution of Dactyloscopy in the United States, with an historical note on the first fingerprint bureau in the United States and a bibliography of personal identification*. Youngstown, Ohio: Beil, 1931.

Federal Bureau of Investigation, *The Science of Fingerprints: Classification and Uses.* Washington, D.C.: Department of Justice, 1985.

Louis Hermann, "Finger Patterns," *American Journal of Police Science,* vol. 2, no. 4 (July–August 1931), pp. 306–10.

B. Laufer, "Concerning the History of Finger-Prints," *Science,* n.s., vol. 45, no. 1169 (May 25, 1917), pp. 504–505.

I. J. Liebenberg, "Obtaining a Print from a Mummified Finger," *Journal of Criminal Law and Criminology,* vol. 41, no. 2 (July–August 1950), pp. 224–25.

Chris C. Plato, "Dermatoglyphics and Flexion Creases of the Cypriots," *American Journal of Physical Anthropology,* vol. 33, no. 3, pp. 421–27.

Cyril John Polson, "Finger Prints and Finger Printing: An Historical Study," *Journal of Criminal Law and Criminology,* vol. 41, no. 4 (November–December 1950), pp. 495–517, and no. 5 (January-February 1951), pp. 690–704.

Chandak Sengoopta, *Imprint of the Raj: How Fingerprinting Was Born in Colonial India.* London: Macmillan, 2003.

Eileen Shorland, "Sir William Jamnes Herschel and the Birth of Fingerprint Identification," *Library Chronicle of the University of Texas at Austin,* vol. 14 (1980), pp. 25–33.

Radhika Singha, "Settle, Mobilize, Verify: Identification Practices in Colonial India," *Studies in History* (India), vol. 16, no. 2 (2000), pp. 153–98.

Karl-Erik Sjöquist and Paul Åström, *Pylos: Palmprints and Palmleaves* (Studies in Mediterranean Archaeology, Pocket-Book no. 31). Göteborg, Sweden: Åströms Forlag, 1985.

George Wilton Wilton, *Fingerprints: History, Law and Romance.* London: W. Hidge, 1938.

24. The signature and handwriting

Béatrice Fraenkel, *La Signature: genèse d'un signe.* Paris: Gallimard, 1992.

Attilio Bartoli Langeli, *Scrittura e parentela: autografia collettiva, scritture personali, rapporti familiari in una fonte italiana quattro-cinquentesca.* Brescia: Grafo, 1989.

Samuel Sams, *A Complete and Universal System of Stenography, or Short-Hand . . . on a plan entirely new, &c.* Bath, Wood & Co., 1812.

Samuel Taylor, *Stenography, or The art of short hand perfected: containing rules and regulations, whereby the most illiterate may acquire the mode of taking down trials, orations, lectures, &c. in a few hours, and be competent by a little experience to practice the same.* Boston: S. G. Snelling, 1810.

John Wilmerding, *Signs of the Artist: Signatures and Self-Expression in American Paintings.* New Haven: Yale University Press, 2003.

25. Gloves

C. Cody Collins, *Love of a Glove: The Romance, Legends, and Fashion History of Gloves, with an Appendix, How to Know Gloves, and How They Are Made*, rev. ed. New York: Fairchild Publishing Company, 1947.

Valerie Cumming, *Gloves*. London: B. T. Batsford, 1982.

B. Eldred Ellis, *Gloves and the Glove Trade*. London and New York: Sir Isaac Pitman & Sons, 1921.

Rudolf Presber et al., *Der Handschuh: Ein Vademecum für Menschen von Geschmack*. Berlin: R. & P. Schaefer, 1914.

Daniel Walter Redmond, "The Leather Glove Industry in the United States." Columbia University Ph.D. dissertation, 1913.

Berent Schwineköper, *Der Handschuh im recht, ämterwesen, brauch und volksglauben* (Neue deutsche Forschungen, 5). Berlin: Junker und Dünnhaupt, 1938.

26. The finger and domestic industry

Clinton G. Gilroy, *The Art of Weaving, by Hand and Power: with an Account of Recent Improvements in the Art, and a Sketch of the History of Its Rise and Progress in Ancient and Modern Times*, 2nd ed. London: Henry Washbourne, 1847.

Marie Girardin et al., *Elegant Work for Delicate Fingers, Consisting of Designs for Crochet Work, Knitting, Netting* ... London: The editor of "Enquire Within upon Everything," 1861.

Markwart Michler, *Die Hand als Werkzeug des Arztes: Eine kurze Geschichte der Palpation von den Anfängen bis zur Gegenwart*. Wiesbaden: Franz Steiner Verlag, 1972.

Azalea Stuart Thorpe and Jack Lenor Larsen, *Elements of Weaving: A Complete Introduction to the Art and Techniques*. Garden City, N.Y.: Doubleday, 1967.

Andrew Wynter, *Subtle Brains and Lissom Fingers: Being Some of the Chisel-marks of Our Industrial and Scientific Progress*. London: Robert Hardwicke, 1863.

27. The finger in drama, music, and dance

Thomas Clayton, "'Fie what a question's that / If thou wert near a lewd interpreter': The Wall Scene in *A Midsummer Night's Dream*," *Shakespeare Studies*, vol. 7 (1974), pp. 101–103.

Clifford Davidson, *Gesture in Medieval Drama and Art*. Kalamazoo: Medieval Institute Publications, Western Michigan University, 2001.

Thomas Elbert et al., "Increased Cortical Representation of the Fingers of the Left Hand in String Players," *Science*, n.s., vol. 270, no. 5234 (October 13, 1995), pp. 305–307.

Bessie Alexander Ficklen, *A Handbook of Fist Puppets*. Philadelphia and New York: J. B. Lippincott Co., 1935.

Charles Maxwell Lancaster, "Gourds and Castanets: The African Finger in Modern Spain and Latin America," *The Journal of Negro History*, vol. 28, no. 1 (January 1943), pp. 73–85.

Nathan Richardson, *Richardson's New Method for the Piano-Forte: An Improvement upon All Other Instruction Books in Progressive Arrangement, Adaptation, and Simplicity*. Boston: Oliver Ditson, 1859.

Richard Charles Shepherd, "The Emergence of a Pivotal Role for the Thumb in Keyboard Fingering during the Early Eighteenth Century and Its Subsequent Impact on Pianistic Idiom." University of Illinois Ph.D. dissertation, 1995.

Fanny de Sivers, "La Main dans la danse européenne," in *La Main* (Eurasie: Cahiers de la Société des Études euro-asiatiques, 4). Paris: Editions L'Harmattan, 1993, pp. 179–88.

Clement Tate, *Digita-Manualis: Tate's Original Method and Exercises for Developing the Flexibility of the Fingers and Wrists, Thereby Overcoming the Chief Difficulties in Playing the Pianoforte, &c., and Securing a Firm and Equal Touch "Without the Aid of Any Instrument."* London: R. Cocks and Co., 1884.

28. The fingers in hand-to-hand combat

John F. Gilbey, *Secret Fighting Arts of the World*. Rutland, Vt.: Charles E. Tuttle & Co., 1963.

Elliott J. Gorn, *The Manly Art: Bare-Knuckle Prize Fighting in America*. Ithaca, N.Y.: Cornell University Press, 1986.

Michael Poliakoff, *Combat Sports in the Ancient World: Competition, Violence, and Culture*. New Haven: Yale University Press, 1987.

Marco Rubboli and Luca Cesari, eds., *L'Arte cavalleresca del combattimento di Filippo Vadi* (15th cent.). Rimini: Il cerchio, 2001.

Hans Talhoffer, *Medieval Combat: A Fifteenth-century Illustrated Manual of Swordfighting and Close-Quarter Combat*, translated by Mark Rector. Mechanicsburg, Pa., and London: Stackpole Books, 2000.

Arthur Wise, *The Art and History of Personal Combat*. Greenwich, Conn.: Arma Press, 1972.

29. Fingers and tobacco

Ludwig Bremer, *Tobacco, Insanity and Nervousness*. St. Louis, Mo.: Meyer Brothers Druggist, 1892.

G. Cabrera Infante, *Holy Smoke*. New York: Harper & Row, 1985.

Iain Gately, *La Diva Nicotina: The Story of How Tobacco Seduced the World*. London: Simon and Schuster, 2001.

Robert S. Gold et al., *Comprehensive Bibliography of Existing Literature on Tobacco*. Dubuque, Iowa: Kendall/Hunt Publishing Co., 1975.

V. G. Kiernan, *Tobacco: A History*. London: Hutchinson Radius, 1991.

Bernard Le Roy and Maurice Szafran, *The Illustrated History of Cigars*. London: Harold Starke, 1993.

William Van Duyn Tobacco Advertisement Collection, 1913–2002, Yale University. New Haven, Conn.: Harvey Cushing/John Hay Whitney Medical Library, MS Coll 20.

Acknowledgments

Apart from a moment of revelation two years ago in the Universitätsbibliothek at the Ruprecht-Karls Universität in Heidelberg, having to do with knuckle hair, all of the research for this book was done either at Yale University in New Haven, Connecticut, or at the British Library and elsewhere in London, and I am grateful to the powerfully learned staffs of those institutions, as well as to my supremely generous colleagues at the Yale Center for British Art, for help of many kinds, particularly from our resourceful head reference librarian, Kraig Binkowski.

During the summer of 2005, I was fortunate to have the assistance of a talented doctoral candidate in Yale's Department of the History of Art, Crawford Alexander Mann III, whom I salute with my right hand, fingers straight, the thumb neatly tucked in. Much of the initial, tedious bibliographical legwork was done by Alex, and I thank him most heartily.

Toward the end of the summer of 2006, it was also my privilege to teach a course alongside Keith E. Wrightson, Randolph W. Townsend, Jr., Professor of History, in the Yale-in-London program at the Paul Mellon Centre for Studies in British Art, our home away from home at 16 Bedford Square. For their generous hospitality I thank my colleagues Professor Brian Allen, Director of Studies; his deputies Frank Salmon, Martin Postle, Kasha Jenkinson; and their staff, but I count it among the greatest strokes of good fortune that I had the privilege of sharing a group of excellent students with Keith Wrightson, and to have had the opportunity to talk with him, then and since, about "micro-history" (of which I am afraid this book is conspicuously not an example; on the contrary), as well as many other things.

A host of other colleagues responded most generously to requests for information and advice, many of them reading and commenting on sections with that unmistakable combination of seriousness, good cheer, and back to seriousness again that characterizes the finest tradition of Yale College: Cassandra Albinson, my associate curator in the paintings and sculpture department, and Mark Aronson, Chief Paintings Conservator, both at the Yale Center for British Art; Edward T. Barnaby, Assistant Dean of the Graduate School of Arts and Sciences; David L. Barquist, now Curator of American Decorative Arts at the Philadelphia Museum of Art; Edward S. Cooke, Jr., Charles F. Montgomery Professor of American Decorative Arts; Helen A. Cooper, Holcombe T. Green Curator of American Paintings and Sculpture (a connoisseur of gloves), and Patricia E. Kane, Friends of American Arts Curator of American Decorative Arts, both of the Yale University Art Gallery; Gary Friedlaender, M.D., Wayne O. Southwick Professor of Orthopedics, Professor of Pathology, and Chair of Orthopedics and Rehabilitation in the School of Medicine; Professor Michael Hatt, now of the University of Warwick; Lawrence Manley, William R. Kenan, Jr., Professor of English; Dale Martin, Woolsey Professor of Religious Studies; Jules David Prown, Paul Mellon Professor Emeritus of the History of Art; Claude Rawson, Maynard Mack Professor of English; Joseph Roach, Charles C. and Dorathea S. Dilley Professor of Theater; William C. Speed of the Department of Genetics; and Barbara Stuart, Lecturer in English.

Colleagues elsewhere were equally generous, especially Steven C. Bullock, Associate Professor of United States History at the Worcester Polytechnic Institute, Worcester, Mass.; Associate Professor Andrew McGowan, Warden of Trinity College in the University of Melbourne; and Sheila M. McIntyre, Associate Professor of History at the State University of New York at Potsdam.

Nor can I fail to pay tribute to certain of my teachers whose great wisdom is occasionally reflected in these pages, though any and all errors of fact are, of course, mine alone: the late Evan L. Burge; Charles R. Curwen, C.V.O., O.B.E., Alison S. Inglis; the late J. Davis McCaughey, A.C., and Jean M. McCaughey, A.O.; Margaret Riddle; Ronald T. Ridley; the late Ian Robertson; Patricia Simons; Geoffrey R. Smith; Daniel Thomas, A.M.; and Chris Wallace-Crabbe.

No doubt specialist reference librarians and archivists are accustomed to receiving unusual requests, but I cannot fail to note the supreme generosity with which the following people responded with great enthusiasm to my especially odd inquiries relating to glove-wearing and nail-polishing habits of the First Ladies: Karen Anson, Archivist, Franklin D. Roosevelt Presidential Library and Museum, Hyde Park, N.Y.; Stephen Plotkin, Reference Archivist, John F. Kennedy Presidential Library and Museum, Boston, Mass.; Helmi Raaska, Archivist, and Nancy Mirshah, Archives Specialist, Gerald R. Ford Presidential Library and Museum, Ann Arbor, Mich.; Albert Nason, Archivist, Jimmy Carter Library and Museum, Atlanta, Ga.; and Jennifer Mandel, Archivist, Ronald Reagan Presidential Library and Foundation, Simi Valley, Calif.

Likewise, I am indebted to Joanna Marschner at Kensington Palace; as always to Pamela Clark, L.V.O., Registrar of the Royal Archives at Windsor Castle, and to the Hon. Lady Roberts, C.V.O., Royal Librarian, for their generous assistance in relation to somewhat vexed questions relating to the Prince Regent's taste in gloves, conventions of court attire at the turn of the last century, and Queen Victoria's sadly undocumented disapproval of nail "polish," *not* varnish (which I suspect may be an unwarranted pink herring). In any case, material in the Royal Archives at Windsor has been quoted with the gracious permission of Her Majesty Queen Elizabeth II. Unfortunately, my carefully worded letters to the Imperial Household Agency in Tokyo, H.H. The Aga Khan, the Chief Justice of the Supreme Court of India in New Delhi, and to the Vatican—relating to various, admittedly arcane points of etiquette, gestures, ring customs, ways with gloves, finger positions, and lore—obviously went astray.

All other permissions to reproduce works of art and acknowledgments of previously published material are credited on pp. xi–xvi and iv, respectively. To the estimable Susan Goldfarb, Debra Helfand, and Georgia Cool at Farrar, Straus and Giroux; to our Bartels Fellow Kara Fiedorek; and to the excellent Andrew Cobb I am grateful for helping me to navigate these and all other shark-infested waters. John McGhee brings the art of copyediting to new heights of sophistication, care, and intelligence.

Halfway through writing this book I had what a good friend of mine described at the time as a biblical experience—seismic, certainly life-changing—a medical emergency from which I have now been mercifully delivered thanks to the expert care of Michael O. Rigsby, M.D. (body), and Helen M. Lankenau, M.D. (mind). These exceptionally difficult circumstances conspired to interrupt the flow, and made it necessary for a time to set my project to one side, and to suspend for the time being various other responsibilities and priorities as well. In the end, I think the book has actually benefited, as I have myself, in many ways.

However, I could not have navigated the unforgettable years of 2006–2009 without the generous and unfailing support of many people to each of whom I owe a special debt of gratitude that is, I fear, larger than I can ever repay—above all, to my remarkable mother, to whose memory the book is dedicated; my three brothers, Nick, Simon, and Hamish, together with their families in Melbourne, Australia; and the following: my curatorial assistant Abigail Armistead, the late John M. Borthwick, Stephen Brady and Peter Stephens, Lucy S. Carruthers and David Jennings, Douglas Chilcott, Deborah Clark, Constance Clement, David C. Cobb, Will Eaves, Helen Endicott, Greg and Andrea Feldman Falcione, Barbara Fargher and the late Philip Fargher, Robert Fellowes, John and Danielle Ginnetti, Fiona Gruber and Mark Williams, Marguerite L. Hancock, Matthew Hargraves, David Alden Heath, Rachel Hellerich, Federay Holmes and Jonathan Jenney, Barry Humphries, C.B.E., Ben Keith and Simon Westcott, Michael Kidd, Thomas E. Lippy, Jr., and David P. Hariton, Geoffrey Little, Patrick McCaughey and Donna Curran, James Magruder, Natasha Maw, Joan Mertens, Michael J. Morand, Brian Porter, Alice and Frank Prochaska, Anne Pye, Geoffrey Quilley and Karyn White, Ron Radford, A.M., David and Deborah Fulton Rau, Kelly and Stuart Read, Peter Rose and Christopher Menz, Fernande E. Ross, Stéphane Roy, Diane Rubeo, Andrew St. John, Professor Emeritus Peter Steele, S.J., Paul Thesinger, Maximilian C. Toth, Cynthia Troup, Cheryl Walters, M.D., Giles Waterfield, Nell White, Nat Williams and Erica Seccombe, Bernard Zirnheld, and, crucially, my old friends Dr. Adam Jenney, of the Alfred Hospital and the University of Melbourne, and Dr. Anne Drake.

My director, Amy Meyers, Adjunct Professor in the Department of the History of Art at Yale, earns a gold star for rare kindness, as do my literary agents, Mary Cunnane, Peter McGuigan, and Natasha Fairweather of the firm of A. P. Watt—indeed, while the seed of the idea for this book was deftly planted long ago in Adelaide by Michael and Janet Hayes, it was brought to germination and safely transplanted by Peter in 2004, and has since then been tended by Mary. My commissioning editor, John Glusman, paid me the compliment of thinking that the idea was good, while Lorin Stein, John's successor as my editor at Farrar, Straus and Giroux, guided it to completion with supreme generosity and esprit de corps. Incidentally, both of these gentlemen have exquisite hands.

Angus Trumble
Yale Center for British Art
New Haven, Connecticut
January 2010

Index

Page numbers in *italics* refer to illustrations.